Embryo as Person

Buddhism, Bioethics and Society

Suwanda H.J. Sugunasiri, *Ph.D.*

Cover: Johnny Osorio

Author photograph: Mo Simpson

Library and Archives Canada Cataloguing in Publication

Sugunasiri, Suwanda H. J.
 Embryo as person : Buddhism, bioethics and society / Suwanda H.J. Sugunasiri.

Includes index.
ISBN 0-9738089-0-X

 1. Bioethics--Religious aspects--Buddhism. 2. Buddhist ethics.
I. Nalanda College of Buddhist Studies II. Title.

BQ4012.S85 2005   **294.3'5694957**   **C2005-902712-6**

Printed and bound at JT Printing, Toronto, Canada

Nalanda College of Buddhist Studies
47 Queen's Park Cres. E.
Toronto, ON M5S 2C3
Canada

in commemoration of

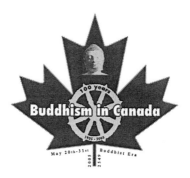

kanadaratthe buddhasaasanassa vassasatam

*100 years since the opening of
the Vancouver Buddhist Church
in 1905*

*25 years since the founding of
the Buddhist Federation of Toronto
in 1980*

*5 years since the founding of
Nalanda College of Buddhist Studies
in 2000*

Toronto, Ontario, Canada
May 20 – 31, 2005

Other Selected Works by Suwanda H. J. Sugunasiri

Buddhism

You're What You Sense: a Buddhianscientific Dialogue on Mindbody, Dehiwala, Sri Lanka: Buddhist Publication Society, 2001

Literature

The Whistling Thorn: An Anthology of South Asian Canadian Fiction, Oakville, ON: Mosaic, 1994

Poetry

The Faces of Galle Face Green, Toronto / Oxford: TSAR, 1995; 2nd edition: Nugegoda, Sri Lanka: Sarasavi Publishers, 2003

Acknowledgements

I wish to acknowledge with thanks that the selections originally appeared in the Toronto Star as follows:
Buddhist Festival a Sumptuous Feast (May 5, 1993); *We All Need to Repay Kindness* (June 11, 1994); *Buddhists Link Karma to Abortion* (Oct. 1, 1994); *There's a Little Piece of Hatred in Every One of Us* (Nov. 26, 1994); *What would Buddha see at General Motors* (March 18, 1995); *Celibacy doesn't guarantee Liberation* (May 6, 1995); *Euthanasia may be a Healing 'Well-death'* (Aug. 19, 1995); *'Soul Myth' Propels Hatred in Us All* (Nov. 4, 1995); *Steering Banks Towards Fairness* (Jan. 13, 1996); *In Death, We're All United* (Feb. 17, 1996); *Buddhist Equinox no Mere Date* (March 23, 1996); *Organ Donors Can Help End 'Religious Killing'* (June 1, 1996); *Dharma Day Message is Moderation* (July 6, 1996); *Meditation Erases Fear of Death* (Aug. 10, 1996); *Time to Include Embryo as Person* (Sept. 14, 1996); *Need Sex, Don't Want it* (Oct. 19, 1996); *An Exercise to overcome Resentment* (Nov. 23, 1996); *Do Celebrate Temple Day* (Dec.28, 1996); *Bare-breast Image Stays in Memory* (Feb. 1, 1997); *Would Euthanasia Hinder Rebirth?* (March 8, 1997); *Cloning not new to Buddha* (April 12, 1997); *Buddha a Good Team Player* (May 24, 1997); *Vacuum mind's over-indulgences* (Aug. 16, 1997); *Buddhist Story puts Death in Perspective* (Nov. 8, 1997); *Ten Paths to Perfection* (Jan. 31, 1998); *Buddhists Keep Faith in Many Cultures* (April, 25, 1998).

CONTENTS

A WORD

My attempt in each of these short pieces is to give the reader a quick glance at the thorny socio-ethical issues of the day, from abortion to homosexuality, from the perspective of the Buddhadhamma (Buddha's Teachings). All but three written for the Toronto Star, they have been pulled together here for the primary reason that there isn't much written in the area, and certainly not within a Canadian context. In putting them together, an attempt has been made to provide some of the contexts the reader may not be familiar with. It is our hope that you will find the material both useful and relevant. Sharing them with others would be a meritorious act.

My thanks go to the Toronto Star for originally publishing the pieces. I thank Jim Vuylsteke for the painstaking editing of the material, and for developing the Glossary and the Index.

The cover is a labour of love by Johnny Osorio whose cheery disposition makes it a pleasure to work with him. Tai Tang, of JTPrinting did an excellent job of printing in a short time.

My wife, Swarna, earns my loving gratitude for living through the immeasurable hours of lost companionship.

Wishing you the best in health and happiness!

In Metta!

Suwanda H. J. Sugunasiri
Nalanda College of Buddhist Studies

May 20, 2005

1

THERE'S A LITTLE PIECE OF HATRED IN EVERY ONE OF US

In a dialogue about the Holocaust with a Jewish scholar, Professor Masao Abe of Purdue University wrote that even though he had no direct or indirect hand in the heart-rending event, he as a Buddhist felt a personal responsibility for it.

His argument was simple. The following little story, well known in Buddhist literature, explains the basis of his stance.

In this story, called *The Jewel Net of Indra,* there is a net that stretches out from the abode of Indra, the lord of gods in popular Buddhism, infinitely, and in all directions.

In each eye of the net is a glittering jewel and, since the net is infinite, the jewels are infinite, too. If we look at any one of them closely, we'll find that all the jewels are reflected in the polished surface of this one jewel. And each of the jewels reflected in this one jewel also reflects all the other jewels.

The essence of the story is that everything in this universe, as physics remind us, is interrelated. So are all human beings, all influencing each other in a myriad of known and unknown ways.

Hate groups, as well as individuals that make up such groups, are part of this gigantic human network. So, just as a close look at a single jewel in Indra's net shows a reflection of all the other jewels, a close look at ourselves will show that each hater, and group, is in each of us! Conversely, in each hater is a part of us.

Is hating the hater then the best response to hate groups?

For one thing, these are our own children. And why are these young minds attracted to such groups? As we hear from defectors, hate groups give them a sense of family, and purpose, if not power. Rock bands give youngsters a collective sense of identity; hate groups recruit new members at such shows.

It is we who have made them feel alienated. We worship the nuclear family and we decimate that, too, when parents decide they have had enough of each other.

Capitalism, which makes our life what it is – comfortable and cosy – makes an idol of individualism as well.

Cut off from relationships, the young become alienated.

We should all, then, feel a sense of responsibility for the birth of hate groups.

It would make sense to work on the enemy within – our anger, hatred, malevolence – before we try to deal with the enemy without.

It is easier said than done, you might say. But there is a way.

We can begin by sending lovingkindness towards ourselves, with the words, "May I be free" as we breathe in, and "from enmity" as we breathe out, followed in succeeding outbreaths with the words "from anger" and "from distress." Finally we wish ourselves: "May I keep myself at peace."

We can direct lovingkindness to a beloved teacher, parents, a dear friend, a neutral person, and finally to "them," our enemy – the hating individuals and the groups that exist around us. This may look like some airy-fairy approach. But the next step is more tangible, seeking to work with hate groups that are now within our thoughts of lovingkindness.

The first step would be to reach out to individuals and leaders among hate groups. Our first contacts perhaps might be a group like SHARP – Skin Heads Against Racial Prejudice[1].

In reaching out, it is important that we listen with honest interest to their genuine concerns. Perhaps we can gain their confidence by inviting them to plan a joint conference to explore the concerns, issues and possible solutions, publicly.

If we are bold, we might even ask to join in celebrating their European heritage week.

With us beside them, the Heritage Front and the National Party of Canada would find it difficult to put Hitler on their posters. We can encourage them to display instead Einstein, John Stuart Mill and Shakespeare.

Working with them is to minimize their alienation. On a more pragmatic level, it is to recognize that, if the hate groups are the problem, they have to be part of the solution.

But most importantly, perhaps, it is also to be concerned with our own well-being and sanity. Specially when, being in Indra's net, our understanding and compassion are their understanding and compassion.

---

1. SHARP, Skin Heads Against Racial Prejudice was an organization created in New York in the late 1980's with the idea of separating the Skinhead movement from the extremist and white-supremacist ideas that it had become associated with. A Toronto chapter was started in 1999.

2

NEED SEX, DON'T WANT IT

Sex is natural and functional, like eating or sleeping, the Buddha would say. From that point of view, a sexual relationship may be explained away as simply two consenting adults giving in to a basic human drive.

But the Buddha also makes a distinction between sex as need and sex as want. If sex as need is what keeps the human (or animal) race going, sex as want is what he explains as passion, one of three desires (or *tanha*) of sentience that keeps each one of us going in the life cycle.

In that light, a sexual act originating in want becomes more than a mere act. "Intent I say is action," says the Buddha. So first of all, sex comes to have karmic consequences, in this life or another, for both man and woman. It can come to be desire leading to more desire or insatiable desire.

If the relationship occurs in the context of a workplace, it comes to be problematic in other ways, too. For starters, there is always the possibility of the partner's own work performance being affected. Possibly, their professionalism may also be compromised. This is why business and industry discourage, or take a serious view of, such relationships.

The relationship may involve unequal partners – say a religious person and congregant, health professional and patient, teacher and pupil, politician and assistant, etc. Then there are other social implications such as abuse of power and the violation of a public trust.

Now if the relationship in that public domain is an extramarital one on the part of one or both partners, then the results may be catastrophic!

First, of course, is the issue of public morality – the example set by people in positions of public accountability. But from a spiritual point of view, the personal morality is surely equally problematic. One has to live with oneself or one's God.

What if, in a relationship developed in a public context, things go sour and one partner's "no" does not mean "no" to the other?

A sign at a Queen's University protest a few years ago read, "Which part of *no* don't you understand?" One might ask the same question of such a person. But would there be a basis for a charge of sexual harassment under criminal law as well?

Now if nary an interest had ever been shown by the offended in a relationship, then, of course, the answer would be clear. It would indeed constitute harassment.

But if the offended had agreed to sex at all, then there is what in Buddhism would be called a "supportive" condition, i.e., encouraging a behaviour (remembering the obvious that without a partner, there would have been no sex).

Sexual passion being the drive it is, and the human being not being a machine, a tap opened is a tap not easily shut off – desire leading to desire. The cells store the pleasure in the memory, and indeed a "no" may even heighten the desire.

"No" after "yes" is, then, not the same as "no" before "yes."

So to speak just in terms of harassment and to ask for the head of an offender would be to go for cold revenge, not justice. It would be worse if no accountability were asked of the offended partner.

The more reasonable and humane expectation would be for both partners to recognize their own contribution to the problem and remove themselves from the environment in which the act flourished.

The responsibility of society would be to insist that both stop pointing fingers or seeking redress, holding both accountable for their behaviour. Not to do this is to send a wrong signal to society, particularly teenagers, that if you can get another in trouble and take revenge, you don't have to take on responsibility.

To allow for a balanced view, by contrast, is to strengthen the foundations of a just society where both women and men begin to treat each other with respect and compassion.

Let us hope that while we continue to think of sex as a healthy need, we will also think through the ramifications of sex as want, at both the personal and the public levels.

3

BUDDHISTS LINK KARMA TO ABORTION

Practically all religions teach about an afterlife.

Buddhism, as does Hinduism, understands this in more tangible terms – rebirth as a human, or animal. Such rebirth is determined by one's karma, the consequences of one's thought and action.

Even though karma and physical rebirth are both beliefs, we don't have to rely entirely on metaphysical teachings.

Contemporary works, such as *Twenty More Cases Suggestive of Rebirth* by Dr. Ian Stevenson in the United States and *Life Between Life* by University of Toronto medical school professor and psychotherapist Joel Whitton, provide intriguing evidence hard to ignore.

Belief or reality, a look at the workings of karma and rebirth may shed some additional light on the abortion debate.

There is no doubt, from the Buddhist point of view, that abortion is killing.

Whether the abortion occurs in the very first week, the first trimester or even after the batting of an eyelid makes no difference. If terminating the life of an interconnected billion cells (this is what a grown-up is) constitutes killing, so does the termination of the single cell about to make such connections.

This fact cannot be taken away even if there are very good practical reasons for an abortion.

Abortion is killing for another reason. It has all five conditions that make up a killing: fact and presence of a living being, knowledge that the being indeed is living, intent to take away life, the act of killing, and an outcome of death.

Karma enters the picture through the condition of intent.

What then would be the karmic resultants of the aborting woman? In this very life, the anguish and the torment, and/or the wrath of the community. Or perhaps a serious accident that would terminate her own life abruptly.

Perhaps the karma would mature only in the next life or down the lane in the wandering wheel of life.

In a sort of tit-for-tat move, would she herself be perhaps aborted? Was that handicapped, blind or mute being that came to be conceived a reckoning of karma? This is certainly not to suggest that all handicaps are karmically conditioned.

Would a more serious consequence be to be born as an animal to be enjoyed, though a chilling thought, by some humans at a feast?

Such are the possible karmic outcomes, of course, not because abortion is any more of a heinous crime than any other killing. They are what awaits any killing.

What seems ironic is that while the father (in the case of rape) may bear the consequences of bringing harm to the woman and to the aborted being, he bears none from an intent to kill. In that sense, abortion may be a second self-victimization for the woman.

If this is how the woman's karma may work, what of the doctor who shared the same intent of killing? Or of the nurses and others who assist?

If the responsibility of laying out the facts with the objectivity of a scientist is the wisdom, the compassion lies in allowing the woman the freedom to make that critical decision.

This is not simply to be fiercely loyal to the independence allowed for by the Buddha's last words, "Be an island unto yourself." It has to do with everybody's karma.

Allowing the woman to reach an informed decision is to help her gain liberational maturity.

But it would also be to work on one's own karma and rebirth toward liberation through the practice of compassion.

So would sitting in meditation with the woman – to provide her with a quietude and mindfulness she desperately needs to manage her karma.

Sending thoughts of compassion to the aborted one would be a final liberational effort.

4

CLONING NOT NEW FOR THE BUDDHA

Had the Buddha been around when the news of the cloning of a sheep hit the wires, he might've simply said, with his usual smile, "What took you so long?"

Not that he provided the technique or predicted the event. But he challenged the scientific community to come up with laboratory evidence for what he had come by in the laboratory of his mind, meditatively, some 2,500 years ago.

What was that? That a human being had nothing that could be called a soul. His teaching was soullessness. And, to show it, he called you and me the "five aggregates."

Your hand touches a hot stove. You feel the sensation. You pull away. And the hand burn becomes part of your memory, and consciousness.

But what is touching? It is bodily contact, and involves many conditions. You have to have a hand; it has to be near the stove; it must not be numb. So, touch is an aggregate.

Touching also results in the aggregate of sensation – again, an aggregate because of its complex conditions. Pulling away is evidence you have perceived danger.

We know that the heat was felt at the fingertip or the skin, but it is also felt in the whole body. The Buddha sees an internal force – an energy force that physically pushes the sensation at the fingers to all over the body. This is the aggregate of force.

The end result is the final aggregate – consciousness, in this case, burn consciousness.

So whatever consciousness each of us has at any given time is the sum total of consciousness that we have built up from the time of conception.

And that's really all that consciousness, the psychological part of our mindbody, is – a complex combination of aggregates and conditions.

In which of the five aggregates is the soul? If the soul is not in the mind, is it perhaps in the body?

Minor problem: each unit of matter that makes up the body, explains the Buddha, is born of consciousness. He calls it a "matter born of consciousness." And our body, again, is one gigantic collection of sense-turned-matter. The hand burn becomes hand-burning consciousness, which, in turn, changes into matter.

If matter that makes up our body is created by the mind in which we found no soul, there obviously cannot be a soul in the body either. So if we can explain both mind and body in terms of conditions, where is the need to look for an outside intervention – the hand of a God?

Dolly the sheep appeared in the universe just fine without the helping hand of God. What this successful cloning showed was that there was nothing in an animal that cannot be explained purely in terms of the process (mind) and structures (body) we call DNA.

If DNA can be replicated by humans working in a lab, where is the hand of God that is said to have created animals?

But, you object: we are human, not animal. True, except that the Buddha puts both animals and humans in the same class.

It would be only a matter of time before we get human cloning. When we have that, our last straw for hanging on to a soul will have vanished. Or will it? Isn't it so comfy and reassuring to have a God around?

5

ORGAN DONORS CAN HELP END "RELIGIOUS KILLING"

Don Cherry[1] is a man with a mission. No, not to promote Hockey Night in Canada, but to promote organ transplants.

Before crisis struck his own family, organ transplant was as close to him as Soviet hockey imports were to the late Harold Ballard[1]! But for Cherry, the need for an organ donor gave new meaning to the dotted line in his driver's license.

Listening to the recent CBC *Metro Morning* interview of Cherry took my mind back a few years, when I was asked to talk in Ottawa at a conference of scientists, medical practitioners and religious leaders from around the world. The organ problem was laid out openly. With advances and successes in transplantation, the demand for organs was sky-rocketing. But religious objection to disturbing body parts in deference to a dead person was choking out the supply, costing savable lives. "Religious killing by withdrawal," someone remarked privately.

So did Buddhism have a view? I was asked to talk about the Buddhist view of the dead.

Labelling any sentient being, i.e., human or animal, a "mindbody," the Buddha points out that what we call the body is, at the most fundamental level, nothing more than bundles of atoms and molecules. In their very nature, they come together and fall apart before we can bat an eyelid. So is the mind energy bundles that also die the moment they are born.

This means, I argued, there is nothing permanent about our minds or bodies. At death, or more accurately at the point of the "exit-mind," what simply happens is that the ever-changing energy leaves the ever-changing body.

Robbed of this "life energy," the poor old body continues to rot away!

So there is no stealing of anybody's anything when an organ, which has lost its mind energy, is severed from a cadaver for transplanting into a living being or for safe-keeping for future use.

What I can now add to all this is that indeed there is some residual energy left in the dead body as, for example, in a light bulb after the switch is turned off, or in a car engine after the key is turned off. (Tibetans, in fact, believe that the mental energy continues for seven days.) Otherwise it could not be transplanted.

But, since leaving untouched whatever residual energy is left is not going to bring back the dead, would not the compassionate thing still be to let whatever body parts that are still pulsating be put to better use, to revitalize a needy body? After all, the exit-mind will do the living for you, in another life.

If I have then convinced you, may I be allowed to make the plea? Would you please consider donating your body parts at death? Many throbbing lives at life's end are waiting – your relatives, neighbours, friends ... and even your enemies. They are inviting you to give life with death. You can use your driver's license or your will.

Now I'm inviting Buddhists, celebrating Wesak[2], the Buddha's birthday, this month (of May), to take the lead and show your true colours of compassion. I, for one, have offered my whole body to science.

I appreciate that we may still have our reservations – religious or otherwise. But if I can hear from you, we might be able to better help make Don Cherry's mission our vision.

1. Don Cherry and Harold Ballard are both Canadian hockey figures. Don Cherry is a hockey broadcaster and commentator. Harold Ballard is the late owner of the Toronto Maple Leafs hockey team.

2. Wesak is the traditional celebration, when Buddhists of all schools and traditions come together to celebrate the Buddha's Birth, (and, in some traditions, Enlightenment and Parinibbana (final demise), as well). It is celebrated on the Full Moon day of May.

6

HOMOSEXUAL MARRIAGE AND BUDDHA DHARMA

So what is the position on homosexual marriage in Buddhism? Well, there is, er, no position!

Let me clarify myself by making a distinction between the *ordained* and the *laity*. If one were to leave the household life to don the yellow robes of a *bhikkhu* (male) or *bhikkhuni* (female), then what is not allowed is not just homosexuality, but any sexuality. Period. No ifs ands or buts. It is not just celibacy either – even masturbation, indeed ejaculation to any extent. Any crossing of the line can be cause for disrobing. The *Vinaya* rules, set out by the Buddha, specifically to govern ordained life, are very clear.

Of course, this strict code has nothing to do with social taboos, but rather that attachment to sexuality, like other attachments (including to oneself), keeps one in the grips of a continuing life cycle of rebirth. And the intended purpose of leaving the household life, of course, is to bring an end to it. To the extent, then, that any kind of indulgence, including even ones like going to a movie, may distract one from the practice, sexuality is taboo for the ordained.

But as for the laity, all the Buddha cautions us, as in the texts, is to watch our sexual *misbehaviour,* this being one of the five self-vows of a Buddhist laity. Adultery, for example, would be a *social* misbehaviour. Forced sex, or unwarranted sexual contact *below the neck and above the knee,* would be others. At a personal level, it could be using an orifice other than the one intended by nature for sexual intercourse.

The operative part is the modifier *mis-*, which clearly

tells us that sex per se is not a sin in Buddha Dharma (Teachings). This can only mean that a sexual relationship between consenting adults is a free choice.

So the issue for the Buddhist is not whether it is homosexuality or heterosexuality, but rather sexuality itself. Or rather mis-sexuality.

A related matter is marriage, which in Buddhism has nothing to do with religion. Since there is no belief in a Creator, marriages are not made in heaven. It is a down-to-earth, civil activity. So, for example, a Buddhist wedding calls for no participation of a clergyman. (But don't be surprised to see one in North America today, or in Japan, it being a cultural practice.) Even registering would be for legal purposes only. A couple may decide on a grand wedding, or a post-nuptial, but again, this would be strictly a social occasion.

Given such an understanding, how does a Buddhist look at homosexuality? One way would be to revisit the institution of marriage itself. Why indeed did the institution of marriage ever emerge? Four reasons come to mind:

- *progeny, to ensure the continuity of the species*
- *providing a stable and healthy environment for the progeny to grow in*
- *keeping the wealth within the family, clan, tribe, ethnic group*
- *human happiness.*

The question then is: to what extent does a homosexual marriage speak to these?

Clearly progeny is no longer an issue today even with heterosexual couples. Some choose not to have children, while others who can't bear children opt to adopt.

There is no reason to believe that providing a healthy environment for children to grow up in is taken any less seriously by homosexual couples.

Wealth sharing is now done in pre-nuptial arrangements, and the law, in any case, does not allow unfair distribution.

Indeed today the glue in two people coming together has come down to the last item: human happiness. If some find it in heterosexuality, it would be difficult to see how it is lost in homosexuality.

Human happiness? Now there is something the Buddha seeks to emphasize – in or outside sexual union. He indeed outlines ways of maximizing human happiness in lay life in fields such as family, economy and polity, without, of course, violating the ethical principles.

So there doesn't seem to be anything in the Buddha Dharma that vitiates against a homosexual union of consenting adults.

Could, then, one in a homosexual relationship be a good Buddhist? Can one keep the self-vows?

How about practicing meditation? Again, can one in a heterosexual relationship practice?

But something the Buddha does emphasize is, "Consider the consequences," personally and socially; homosexual or heterosexual. That is to say that, after the cheering is over, be mindful of the implications, and complications, of union: responsibility, spousal abuse, messy divorce, and legal wranglings to share the wealth.

Finally, there is nothing to say that a tradition of 2500 years, and cultural norms, may not have a louder voice in the debate than the Dharma itself.

7

"SOUL MYTH" PROPELS HATRED IN US ALL

Turning suffering on its head is a well-known Buddhist axiom. So even though we don't want to hear one more word about Paul Bernardo[1], he provides us with a wonderful opportunity to reflect upon our own behaviour.

Take, for example, his raping of Leslie Mahaffy and Kristen French. Lust, albeit in its extreme form, motivates it, we would all agree. But the Buddhist viewpoint would say that behind the lust is something more – the general category called *greed*.

And all of us are greedy for something or other. If a child is greedy for a candy bar, we adults are greedy for the dollar. Or for that new car, that promotion, that fame, that power, that new hairstyle, that perfume.

But our greed doesn't end there. Like Bernardo, we are greedy for love, and sex as well. But unlike Bernardo, our greed is for the ordinary, healthy sex, needed for the continuation of the species. And also for the love needed to maintain relationships. Nevertheless, however normal all these desires may be, they would be fueled by greed.

Bernardo was also convicted of killing these young women. If a killing were associated with lust, and hence greed, it would fall under the general category of hatred in the Buddhist understanding.

If we reminded ourselves that the more common face of hatred is anger, then we know right away that we all feel it, too. Not just Bernardo or Karla Homolka, or prison inmates.

The Buddha sees these two, greed and hatred, in the

company of another, *delusion*. Thinking that I am the best in the crowd, or that the world will end in the not-too-distant future may all be examples. But here he is talking of a more fundamental delusion – that there is something unchanging, permanent, called the "soul."

We don't need sociology to know that society changes. Science tells us that by the time you have finished reading this column, you will have replaced a few million cells. Your order for cells for a whole new skeleton will take only a few months! And the Buddha calculates that the mind goes down the tube (if only to re-emerge) 17 times faster than the body!

If we now convince ourselves that not just the body, but the total "mindbody" is "born, comes to be and passes away," as the Buddha says, we still somehow seem to shy away from the logical conclusion – if everything changes, how can there be anything that doesn't change?

We can also ask where exactly this unchanging soul we delude ourselves to believe in hangs its hat. It cannot be in the mind, which, as we have just seen, changes.

The Buddha pointedly asks if the soul we delude ourselves about is in the sensations. If so, in which of the sensations – happy, unhappy or neutral? And what would we have to say when a happy sensation gives way to an unhappy one? That the soul has just died and was born again?

It would not be too long after this, one would think, before we begin to wonder if the idea of a soul is, in fact, not a figment of our imagination, a defense mechanism to assure ourselves that the continuous change does not sweep us off our feet? Our belief in a soul, however, is apparently so cast in iron that logic goes cold at the touch! Indeed to make it palatable, we call it "self" and "ego" in psychological language.

And so, from a Buddhist point of view, it can be said

that it is this "soul myth" that propels people like Bernardo and Homolka, and you and me, into our greed and hatred.

Bernardo went overboard, assisted by a porn industry, film industry and a society that is also deluded into believing in a permanent soul. So are we.

We too can live our ordinary lives believing in a soul. Millions do. But one preventive measure we can take to minimize the possibility of our hatred and greed growing into a monster is to take some time to think of what fuels them. If this leads to a questioning of reality as we know it, the Buddha would offer as alternative his teaching of *anatta* "asoulity,"[2] linked to the other understanding of impermanence, to consider.

He would only ask you not to take his word for it, but to see for yourself. He would offer meditation as the lab in which to do the experimenting.

---

1. Paul Bernardo was convicted for kidnapping, brutalizing and then killing two teenage women in the late 1980s. At the time, the case received an immense amount of publicity.

2. *Asoulity*: this term, which replaces the more traditional term, *soullessness*, or *selflessness*, seeks to capture the original sense of the Pali term *anatta*, made up of, *atta*, "soul," plus *a[n]-*, absence/negation, to suggest the absence of any reality called the soul. Asoulity is modelled after *amorality* as contrasted with *immorality*.

8

CELIBACY DOESN'T GUARANTEE LIBERATION

Has celibacy got anything to do with spirituality and liberation? The question has become as pressing to Buddhism in North America as it is to Catholicism.

We, of course, know that the Buddha practiced celibacy even before he became Enlightened. In fact, leaving his wife (and son and palace) signified the beginning of his very spiritual search. His earliest disciples, both men and women, practiced it, too, as do many serious practitioners around the world today.

But in North America, just as many, and perhaps even more, do not. This includes not only an increasing number of lay practitioners of meditation but respected teachers, too, immigrant or new Buddhist, with large followings.

So where does celibacy stand in Buddhism?

To begin with – take a sigh – sex in Buddhism isn't a "sin," and, with no God to supervise behaviour, certainly not a "punishable offense." Sex is, shall we say, like food – no more, no less. If you have it to sustain yourself (i.e., as an outlet of sexual energy), to maintain relationships, to bring forth progeny, and the like, it'll do you good. But if you over-indulge, it stings you, just as if you overeat you'll throw up. It can ruin your health and wealth, bring unhappiness, end marriages, ruin families, and dare I say society?

All that the Buddhist precept relating to sex (one of five basic precepts) calls for is "avoidance of *mis*behaviour in sex." Just as the one relating to intoxicants reminds one to avoid the stage beyond which "one's consciousness is *altered*."

But craving for sex does fall under the category of "attachment." Just as food and liquor do, or even a car, a Bach concerto or a painting by Renoir. The Buddha's second Noble Truth is that we continue in our life cycle of *samsara* (put another way, are born again and again) because of attachment. Not just in sex, but in all our senses. Craving for sex, like food or liquor, then, is a bodily attachment.

But it is an attachment in the mind too. "Mind is forerunner," says a line in the *Dhammapada*, a book of verses that contain the quintessence of Buddhist thought[1].

The problem in sex for the Buddhist practitioner, then, is that because of its pervasive nature, its potent power to keep one in attachment, it can serve as a way of keeping the mind stuck on it.

Again, like any other attachment, a mind stuck on sex is a mind unavailable to see things clearly. But again, no more, no less than a mind stuck on anything else – taking life; taking what is not given; speaking falsehoods and backbiting, slandering and the like; and taking liquor to excess (to bring to mind the other four basic precepts).

So sex in Buddhism is not the pits. It is just one among the many attachments. But it is not to be reified either. The best Buddhist argument for celibacy, then, perhaps is that it can facilitate our getting rid of another of the many conditions that keeps us in attachment.

But can a person attached to sex advance spiritually? Can one build a wall standing on the first rung of a ladder? Of course. While the level of the wall built from the first rung is not the end point, the rest of the wall cannot come to be without the foundation of this lower level.

No doubt we will have to polish the idea to match the Buddhist understanding, but the practice of meditation is sort of like building a wall. One brick at a time ... It is such an understanding that allows the North American practitioner to be both in lay life and in the spiritual life at the same time.

But can one come to the final liberation of *nibbana/nirvana* in the heat of sex? This is a moot point hotly debated in Buddhist circles.

But all Buddhists would agree on one thing. While celibacy is not the last resort of the scoundrel, it doesn't guarantee liberation either!

---

1. There are a number of translations of the *Dhammapada* available in the market, e.g., Cleary 1994, Narada, 2001.

9

TIME TO INCLUDE EMBRYO AS PERSON

One day last month, I planted a small piece of rock, shining and beautiful, in potting soil, watered it and kept it in the sun. I have been going out to look at it since then, but have never been able to see it sprout into a sapling!

What a dumbhead, you say, pointing out that, of course, you can't get a rock to grow! Indeed I now remember the excitement as a kid when a bean seed I had planted as part of a biology experiment in school, sprouted within a few days. I had placed cow-dung in the pot, watered it and kept it out in the sun.

The seed sprouted because there were suitable conditions. But the rock did not, though under the same conditions. Which goes to show that for life to emerge, there has to be not only conditions, but an inherent *potential* as well. Which also means that life must be considered to begin long before the stem and the leaves begin to grow.

These thoughts have begun to run through my mind in the context of several issues that have hit the headlines recently – health professionals trying to decide the fate of frozen sperm samples after five years; a mother wanting to abort one of her twin fetuses; another shooting her unborn child; a judge ordering a pregnant woman to take treatment for her drug-addiction. The basic issue at the back of all these seems to be, "What constitutes a 'person'?"

We have to be careful here. The term "person" is not one but two concepts. There is the ordinary meaning when we refer to a woman, man or child, as in "S/he is a bad person." It refers to one's humanness.

Then there is the other, legal one, associated also with power and rights. It still refers to humanness, but by arbitrary definition only. So, at one time, e.g., women were not persons, a fate pushed upon blacks, Jews, untouchables, gypsies, native people, etc. in different lands in different times.

Mixing up the two meanings – law and reality – seems to be what is clouding the issue.

Legal principles, practices and procedures, we may want to remind ourselves, evolve on the basis of the understanding legal professionals bring to their work of nature, and society. If our analysis of nature and society is faulty, then the law will reflect that too.

Which is how the particular groups came to be depersonalized, and ... dehumanized. It is our increasingly more accurate understanding that eventually led, or will hopefully lead, to the inclusion of such groups under the rubric of "person."

But today the fetus and the embryo still await inclusion, as if having to prove they are not rocks but seeds, with every potential to grow into what one is at birth – with functional organs and limbs. The difference between the born and the unborn is a matter of degree rather than content, i.e., what goes into making them. Take, for example, the baby one split second before birth. While we call this life form a "fetus," he or she has everything a newborn has – limbs and senses. The one difference is that his or her breathing is not associated with the air outside. Inside the womb, life's movements go on – kicking, eyelid batting, feeling heat and cold, being happy and agitated, brain activity.

And, of course, the physical limbs begin to appear long before that split second before birth – first, traces of hands and legs in the fifth week, the heart in the fourth, the rudimentary heart and brain in the second, etc. When we consider that it takes a fertilized ovum from five to six days to reach the uterus – we cannot but say that life as a human has indeed begun, even as it enters the uterus.

But what about that first week? What is it that makes the trip to the uterus? It is nothing but the very first cell, dividing itself and forming into an increasing number of cells, hanging together. Is that not human life? Come to think of it, aren't our legs, hands, head – indeed the whole mindbody – also clumps of cells hanging together?

And that goes for our minds, too. Another word for "mind" is "consciousness," which in the Buddha's understanding, is the outcome of a stimulus, or input, interacting with the ongoing life energy in 17 stages. Since the very first instant of life is called "conception consciousness," then the very first cell that results from the fertilization of the ovum must also, by definition, have exactly the same mental *process* (not the content) of the consciousness that you and I experience this very moment. There may be a measurable difference between the body parts of a born one and an unborn one; but not when it comes to consciousness.

If that be the case, then, on every rational and scientific basis, we cannot help say that what we have at the point of conception is indeed human life, the same as we have up to death. What is missing are, of course, the two elements: limbs and functionality. If we were to say that the first cell at conception, or the multiple cells in its first week in the uterus that do not yet show such functional limbs, do not constitute human life, I can see ourselves getting into an uncomfortable contradiction. It would be the same thing as saying that one who is not fully functional (e.g., a handicapped person) is less than human! A person in a coma would be only one-sixth human, since only his mind-sense, the sixth sense in Buddhism, is functional.

Returning now to the four issues that triggered these thoughts, the matter of sperm samples can be easily dealt with. There is no *new* life involved, so it entails no termination of life. The aborting of the unborn twin, however, does. The decision to abort may be medical, and justified, but it has to be with the understanding that it is a human that is being killed. To equate the natural death of a fertilized egg, like the natural death after birth, with the intentional killing entailed in abortion would be to confuse the issue.

As to the mother who shot the fetus, it would not only be immoral but would also have serious social repercussions for the law to accept an argument that the unborn is not a person and therefore the act of shooting a fetus does not constitute killing, nay, first degree murder. It would also be allowing itself to continue to live in the speculative, religious and philosophical but unscientific past. If it wishes to come to the twenty-first century, as it must, it must immediately look to the scientific knowledge available, and change the law to recognize humanness from the very first mind-moment of conception. If it cannot come fast enough, should we encourage judges to force its hand by beginning to break the law by ruling that the mother who shot her baby is guilty of murder?

10

VACUUM MIND'S OVERINDULGENCES

Vacuumed your mind lately? Summer is a good time to do it.

For a whole year, we look forward to that great two-week getaway. We sunbathe, splash, eat, engage in a lot of sex, sightsee, play sports.

These are all great activities. But they are also ways of piling up sensual garbage. No, I don't mean sexual. I mean garbage collected in the six bins of eye-sense, ear-sense, nose-sense, tongue-sense, body-sense and mind-sense.

No nonsense this business of garbage collecting. Our very life depends on it. Our senses would be starved without all this "contact food," as the Buddha calls it. And, specifically in relation to the mind sense, "consciousness food" and "volitional food." Whenever we lie on the beach and let the sun's rays soothe us, we're enjoying our contact food of the day through touch or the body-sense. The same when we see a gorgeous waterfall, this through our eyes.

When we see a robust beauty or a shapely hunk and lust after her or him, we have been served up a dish of volitional food. Not content with merely taking in the figure objectively (contact food), we've made a decision to have some of it for ourselves.

When we recreate in memory the great time we had playing beach ball, we're bringing in the tray of consciousness food. The game was real; we did it. But the replay is something we have recreated in our mind.

So, it's not only the Buddha's fourth nutriment of "solid food" we buy at the supermarket that we need for our survival.

But needing is one thing and wanting another. That is where the piling up of garbage begins, from the time of conception. During our vacations, we accumulate it with a vengeance to make up for the over-indulgence denied us over fifty weeks.

That is why we need some summer vacuuming. Let us go to the door of our mind and see who has gone in and out of it over the last, say, one week. Looking for some frequent visitors, see if anger has gone through it. Then ask what made the visitor go past that; was it anything I did or was it something somebody else did?

The next logical questions would be why and how. What was it that allowed the visitor through the door? What might I have done differently to stop him or her?

Push it back to the last one year, since your last vacation. If necessary, take a week, month, season at a time. Then, do the same thing with the other two frequent-flier visitors – stupidity and sensuality.

Now we go to the other two doors: word and body, and go through the same process.

Once we have sucked out the dirt, we can explore what kind of antidotes to anger, stupidity and sensuality we would like to send out through our doors.

How about friendliness, wisdom and self-restraint for starters? I am sure you can come up with others. What language, thoughts, body signals should we encourage?

We can do this in relation to those persons who went past the doors. Or we can do it in relation to the family circle of friends and colleagues. Visualize the person.

So let us take out our vacuum cleaners this summer.

And if we now watched our doors over the next one year, again taking an hour, day, week, at a time, we won't have to spend as much time vacuuming next summer. We can put the saved-up time and energy to better use cultivating our critical compassion.

11

BUDDHIST FESTIVAL A SUMPTUOUS FEAST FOR HUNGRY SPIRITS

Some restaurants in Toronto offer "Buddha delight soup." But if you want a real taste of what the Buddha provides, you should visit one of the 25[1] or so temples in and around Metro Toronto this month.

Beginning with the full moon tomorrow[2], and every Saturday and/or Sunday in May, the more than 87,000 Buddhists in the city will be commemorating Wesak, the triple celebration of the Buddha's Birth, Enlightenment and Final Demise (Parinirvana).

When Prince Siddhartha was born to Queen Mahamaya and King Suddhodana some 2,537 years ago, a royal sage predicted he would be either a universal monarch or a Buddha. The king – surprise, surprise – made sure the growing prince experienced all the worldly attractions, from an excellent education to sports to wine and women, eventually marrying him off to his cousin, Yasodhara, at 16.

But the spiritual yearnings rumbling within Siddhartha were too overpowering to keep him in the royal household. On a moonlit night at the age of twenty-nine, he left to look for something called Nirvana, a peaceful, pure and deathless state.

Going to all of the renowned teachers, he soon mastered the major trick of the trade: meditation. Each teacher offered him co-leadership, but not seeing the way to Nirvana, he left all of them to take up a solitary sojourn of six years.

He even did something quite foolish. Having come from a life of luxury and indulgence, he began to think that perhaps it was the appetites of the body that got in the way of Enlightenment. So he denied himself even food and water – and nearly died.

This experience, however, provided a practical insight – the wisdom of avoiding extremes. Returning to a saner lifestyle, he continued his search for Nirvana, all the while fine-tuning his research tool, the mind. And one day, as he sat under a tree – today we know it as the Bodhi tree – he resolved never to rise until insight dawned upon him. Soon enough, he experienced the Awakening.

What was this great insight? Nothing much, really, when you come to think of it – simply that suffering (*dukkha*) is the reality of life. Why? Because we are stuck, like Krazy Glue, on ourselves, the things of the world, our happiness and unhappiness, our life and even our death. Or on nirvana itself, that elusive final goal.

But how does one free oneself from self-centredness in order to experience Nirvana? That's easy, the Buddha seemed to say: "Follow the Path," the Fourth Truth. He insisted you didn't have to take his word for it: "Come and see," he said.

Which is what keeps me in Buddhism. When I sit in meditation and visualize myself to be a dead body that in time decays and eventually turns into dust, I need no Buddha, nor modern science, to tell me that things "come to be and pass away." I can see no static, unchanging soul.

It is to encourage such personal realization that the Buddha advised against accepting anything, even his own words, without a test.

But if I need guidance, I am not left in an ethical vacuum. In one of the spokes of the Noble Eightfold Path there is Excellent Behaviour, which includes friendliness, compassion, altruistic joy in sharing, pleasant language, equality and promotion of the over-all social good.

And when I am faced with modern issues, it is comforting to realize that the Buddha has already been there.

He bucked tradition by admitting women to the order.

He showed regard for the environment by laying down detailed instructions to his disciples for the construction of outdoor toilets and forbade even snipping leaves off plants.

Most important, there is not one word or act of the Buddha that can be quoted or used as an excuse for aggression of any kind.

It is such a sumptuous menu of compassion and wisdom, realizable by one and all through calm perseverance, that the temples and Buddhist community – Chinese, Vietnamese, Japanese, Korean, Laotian, Cambodian, Burmese, Indian, Sinhalese (Sri Lankan) and Western, among others – will be serving this month.

If meditation whets your appetite, then any temple would do.

If however, you want to mingle with the largest community, then the Chinese Cham Shan Temple would be your fare.

A fully ordained Western woman teacher will welcome you at Tengye Ling Tibetan Centre.

If you want a full day of Zen meditation, art, music and discussion, the Buddhist Temple on Vaughan Rd.[3] is the obvious choice.

If you're looking to meet all types of Buddhists under one roof, then come to Rosedale Heights School May 29 for an international menu of religious practices and cultural performances.

You might even get a taste of real ethnic food that beats "Buddha delight soup" hands down.

1. Now over seventy. See www.buddhismcanada.com for details.
2. Written for the month of May, 1993
3. The Zen Buddhist temple has since moved from this location.

12

FULL HOUSING THROUGH HOMELESSNESS

"Homelessness" is a good Buddhist virtue. It means leaving the home literally, to live outdoors or in a meditation hut, to take to a life of simplicity.

Like Prince Siddhartha, the future Buddha, did.

But, of course, we can't possibly leave our homes to live outdoors. We need a roof over our heads, certainly with our Canadian winters.

"Homelessness," however, is something we can all cherish even as we continue to enjoy living in our homes.

That is, if we thought of it as an attitude, a mind-set.

Throughout history, many a prince and princess, of all faiths, have taken to this voluntary homelessness. They have moved from home to house, where the walls and the roof are simply a convenience, to practice the virtuous life.

They have rediscovered the original house – literally a roof over their heads.

Most of us others in society, however, have come a long way from looking at a house simply as some mortar and wood put together to meet a basic need.

Today, a house is not only a home, but an extension of our ego. So the bigger the house, the higher our egos fly.

Pandering to the ego, the industry advertises the size of the master – oops! – main bedroom, and the number of washrooms. And, of course, the lot size.

Location, location, location, the industry also reminds us. Not necessarily for its good neighbours, but for the real estate value.

So the home becomes our castle – in the literal sense of a status symbol.

Our home, or not having one, locks us into a caste system. The Brahmins in the single houses in Toronto's upscale Rosedale and Forest Hill, and the untouchables in subsidized row housing! Or no housing.

The Brahmin egos begin to compete internationally when developers remind us that the price per square foot in prime Toronto is a mere fraction of that of London, New York or Tokyo. So Hong Kong money pours in, making the competition literally international. The result? The housing crisis.

It is our own and the industry's greed that have created the problem.

And we and the industry alone can solve it. Cooperatively.

Governments can only help.

The antidote to our greed and bloated egos is the attitude of homelessness. We need to develop the mind set that would allow us to rediscover the home as house – and let go of it as part of our ego.

Yes, we need a comfortable home to come to after a hard day's work.

Yes, a house makes more money than we ourselves do even as it sits idly, not moving a limb, as Gary Lautens[1] caricatured in a recent column!

Yes, a house is an investment hedge and a future investment.

But a homelessness mind-set can make that investment available to all.

By helping us put things in perspective.

By helping us see how we have created it for ourselves.

By helping us go to the roots of the problem, and deflate our egos, and cool the greed.

By making our ears sensitive to the cries of the new

house-poor, the middle class professionals.

By putting some compassion back into our lives.

To expect the industry to develop a homelessness mind-set might need legislative help from governments.

Should the government bring industry under conflict of interest and insider trading legislation? After all, an "affordable house" in Toronto jumped nearly fifty percent in a matter of few days when it was bought and resold by a real estate agent.

Should the government view comparing Toronto prices to prices elsewhere as inflationary advertising which invites price galloping and bring in advertising standards legislation? As done for the tobacco industry?

Should builders be required to apportion their projects – 25% low cost housing, 25% luxury housing, and the balance average housing?

Of course, a homelessness mind-set can help the industry legislate itself. Like other professional groups do.

A homelessness mind-set might not solve the housing crisis immediately. But in the long run, it can lead to affordable housing for all of us.

And we will also have rediscovered the role of philosophy in our lives. That when everything else fails, philosophy kicks in!

When a little philosophy gets into action, maybe issues of abortion, poverty, education, crime and so on might benefit as well.

The winter of our minds – cold, uncaring, cruel and grueling – is not what we Canadians take pride in.

Our tradition of compassion should naturally turn us to the spring of the mind : homelessness!

---

1. Gary Lautens was a humour columnist in the Toronto Star.

13

BUDDHIST EQUINOX NO MERE DATE

Ohigon. Spring *Ohigon!*

March 21 is just another date on our calendar ... officially spring but still too cold for comfort. But for the Japanese, like those who come to the Toronto Buddhist Church the Sunday closest to the equinox, it is time for celebration.

The day begins with the family Sunday service. Congregants sit in the pew, as in a church, to background organ music. The minister, or *sensei*, leads. A large scroll hangs beside the pulpit, the words, *Namo Amida Butsu*, meaning "Homage to the Buddha," written in bold characters, top to bottom, Japanese style.

Service over, the congregants walk over to the basement for a luncheon of yummies for my tummy.

But now begins the *Keiro Kai*, the Seniors' Appreciation Event. If you've turned 77 ("double joy," Izumi Sensei explains) or 88 ("fulfilment and prosperity, for that is how long it takes for a rice seed to mature"), a medal recognizes you. Fun follows, with *Odori* folk dances, singing, music and, of course, that truly national game, bingo!

But why all this celebration?

Equinox, as the term reminds us, means "equal night," and, of course, also "equal day." But the Japanese, Korean and Tibetan Buddhists in particular see a much deeper symbolism than mere measurement in the equinox. For them, nature's equilibrium stands for the Buddha's Middle Path. So it is a chance to go to the "respectful other shore" (what *o-hi-gon* means) of liberation.

We know that Siddhartha Gautama (later, the Buddha)

came from a princely, dare I say filthy rich, life of extreme indulgence – literally of wine and women. In search of liberation, he then went to the other extreme: asceticism. Surviving on the barest, he even tries to stop his breathing completely.

The near-death experience is enough to drive some sense into him, and return him to the fold of ordinary living. Eschewing the extremes now, he arrives at the principle of the Middle Path, experientially. This principle also becomes the central pillar of his teachings in the form of the Noble Eightfold Path.

Nothing fancy, y'know, about the eight spokes of the wheel, as the Path is often called. One can begin with any of them – either listing them or trying to practice them. But let us begin with *concentration*, in the quiet of our home, early morning, at bedtime or when the kids are out playing. How about concentrating on your breath, focusing on the tip of your nose?

The last time you concentrated on a math or business or family problem, a focusing of the mind came upon you. This the Buddhists call *mindfulness*. It is maintained only with *effort*.

Obviously living a life of concentration and mindfulness, every minute of every day, can only be an ideal. In everyday life, people have to make a living, engage in other activities, talk, think and the like. So the Path calls attention to these as well. In relation to *livelihood*, for example, this means asking ourselves whether bearing arms, selling meat, hunting animals or selling your body constitutes excellence in living.

For it is excellence that the Middle Path calls for.

Continuing the wheel, we arrive at Excellent *Action, Speech, Thought* and *Understanding*. But what does "excellent" mean here? Think of the taut string of a finely tuned musical instrument, the Buddha explains – not too loose, not too tight!

The Middle Path, then, means not overdoing, and doing everything in balance. So meditating all day, and getting stoned at a bar in the evening, is not to practice the Middle Path. Talking sweetly while harbouring thoughts of ill-will (sounds familiar?) isn't either.

It is this balance that the Japanese and other Buddhists reflect upon and celebrate as *Ohigon*.

Can I then invite you to join the spirit of *Ohigon*, by wearing a cheery smile on your face as you go to work, tomorrow and the rest of the month until spring does arrive? If you want it to come from deeper within, you might consider practicing mindfulness.

Let a hundred smiles bloom, to blow away the winter blahs!

14

STEERING BANKS TOWARD FAIRNESS

Allelujah to our banks! Creating wealth is what a capitalist system is all about – making a bigger pie available for our roads, hospitals, airports, healthcare, education and our general standard of living. Their billion-dollar profits are a shining example.

But creating wealth does not just happen. There has to be a human being behind it. So I would not grudge the bank managers their salaries and bonuses.

To scream my head off just because I am not a direct beneficiary of their success story would be sheer hypocrisy, jealousy and enmity, none of which, the Buddha says, are conducive to liberation.

The Buddha recognizes the importance of creating wealth, and protecting it. He even gives tips on how to do them well!

But his advice to millionaires was not any different from that to the average Joe and Jane. "Excellent Livelihood" is making a living in such a manner that brings happiness to oneself but no harm to others.

Applied to the banks, what then might constitute Excellent Livelihood?

Looking after one's employees has to be at the top. Developing a work structure to facilitate working moms and dads to spend more time with their children, for example.

If the Royal Bank and the others absolutely have to let employees go, building strategies for their continued sustenance into the severance package would constitute bringing no harm to those who have devoted a good part of their lives helping make the profits.

Bank charges have become the cash cow of the

industry. Many, no doubt, are justified. But there is something unexcellent about charging for withdrawing one's own money. And for having an account? C'mon!

After all, bank profits come partly from investments, and it is our money that is invested. So why shouldn't we be paid reasonable interest? Excellent Livelihood would mean treating account holders as shareholders, worthy of a fair dividend.

Banks would still have the money, but not through punishment but rather positive reinforcement. It would constitute not bringing harm to customers.

In case you think this a loony idea, let me take you back to Tangalla, my town in Sri Lanka. The co-op shop made profits by selling us all our needs, from clothing to food. But at the end of the year, we lined up to get our share of the profit – based on purchases.

Finally taxes. It would be practicing Excellent Livelihood for the banks, instead of finding loopholes to avoid taxes, to pay their fair share toward the continuing working of capitalism.

If banks were to compete with each other to be the best example of Excellent Livelihood, they would get to eat the cake (make money) and keep it (make customers happy). They would be helping to create a society that is both humane and wealth-creating.

Since Excellent Livelihood is a spoke in the Buddha's Noble Eightfold Path, who knows, bank bosses and managers may even be facilitating their own spiritual liberation!

15

BUDDHA A GOOD TEAM PLAYER

I got a call recently about a citizen of the world on the Ottawa Senators hockey team – the Buddha. What did I think of the team's good-luck charm Buddha, the reporter wanted to know.

I said that I had read with amusement that the team now had "a twenty-fifth man on their roster – a carved Buddha that has been the team's good-luck charm on their march to the playoffs." A photo of a standing pot-bellied laughing figure carried the caption, "Sens' secret weapon?"

Gimme a break! Good-luck charm? Buddha? What's going on here?

"Buddha power" – as in the "cheer cards" given to the fans – seems to have worked to bring the Senators into the playoffs, even though they collapsed under the weight of the Buffalo Sabres.

The Buddha must be thrilled to pieces, I am sure, that he wields such power. If that means he somehow magically gets into each player on ice, orchestrating the positioning, passing, shooting and goaltending, you can forget it. That's to turn the Buddha into some all-powerful God. But none such exists, the Buddha has asserted.

But if Buddha Power is the confidence the team has garnered through such belief, then that is a possibility. What does the trick, of course, is not some external hand but the re-energizing of the power within each of us, focused as never before.

Focus – now that is a word the Buddha can identify with. It is billed "Right Mindfulness" and "Right Concentration" in his Noble Eightfold Path.

The Chicago Bulls apparently discovered it several seasons ago. Manager Phil Jackson, a Zen practitioner of more than twenty years, not only teaches his players to experience "the joy of being in the moment" but also "to blend their individual talents with the consciousness of the group." Players centre on selfless teamwork and, as Jackson puts it in *Tricycle* (Summer 1994), the leading popular Buddhist journal, "aggressiveness without anger."

Judging by the Bulls' impressive record, it works wonders. Awareness and teamwork, not dumb luck, that is.

For US triathlete Paula Newby-Fraser, concentration is in movement. "I do daily moving meditation" she says in *Tricycle* (Summer, 1995). "Being in my body completely as I run is a deep practice for me. It is the Buddhist teaching of balance, the middle path, that means the most to me."

Respected Senators, then, keep your pot-bellied figure, even if it is not, in fact, the Buddha, but a Chinese sage of anonymity. Not for charm, dumb luck or Buddha Power, but just as a reminder.

Let his nose remind you to be mindful of your breathing meditation, and the eyes to be vigilant about teamwork. The pot-belly should surely remind you to cut out the fat!

But win or lose, you are sure to grow in your spiritual life.

And if you want to experience the Buddhist variety, come down to Nathan Philips Square June 7[1] for the Buddhist Celebration for Canada and World Peace, where you will find a lot of Buddha Power. The participants will have just spent May, full moon to full moon, celebrating the Buddha's Birth, Enlightenment and Final Demise (Parinirvana).

1. The reference is to year 1997.

16

BUDDHISTS KEEP FAITH IN MANY CULTURES

"Buddhish" was what a Jewish colleague of mine was called when he embraced Buddhism. It was apparent to users of that name that something of Jewishness remained.

My colleague – as do many other Ju-Bu's as they are sometimes fondly called – encourages and joins in the *Bar-* and *Bat-mitzvahs*[1] of his children, keeps a *menorah*[2] at home and celebrates Jewish holidays with his Jewish wife and children.

But becoming Buddhist to him means that these have lost their religious significance. So, he can be said to have retained his Jewishness only culturally.

There is nothing unusual or original about separating the religious from the cultural. Many Chinese Buddhists, for example, may be religiously Buddhist, but culturally they are every bit Chinese. By that I mean they retain much of their homegrown Taoist and Confucian practices and beliefs.

North American Christians who have become Buddhist – more than a million of them – also retain much of the Western culture and ethos that has evolved within the context of Christianity.

Each of the several Buddhist communities that lives in Canada likewise can be said to be culturally Vietnamese or Burmese or Sinhalese or Japanese, but still be Buddhist.

So, how do you identify a Buddhist?

Growing up in Sri Lanka as a Sinhalese Buddhist, I had always thought that to be Buddhist is merely to keep to my training principles: abstaining from killing, stealing, inappropriate sexual behaviour, lying and slandering, and taking intoxicants to an extent that would alter my consciousness.

Then, the North American Buddhists I met defined their Buddhistness in terms of meditation only – gazing at a wall twenty-four hours a day, as we teased.

Then, there are the Tibetan Buddhists who believe in magic and oracles and engage in Tantric sex. Japanese *Jodo Shinshu* Buddhists invoke the name of the Buddha so they will end up in Heaven *Sukhavati*, a blissful place not very different from the Christian heaven.

So which of these various Buddhists are Buddhists?

Clearly all of them are. The Buddha only asks you to "come and see" for yourself. But he knows that the way he is understood and his teachings practiced is going to be different from person to person, culture to culture, time to time. Not that his teachings are relative, but that everyone's understanding will be.

So, is it that anybody can claim to be a Buddhist?

Just about. You have only to put a tag on yourself.

But I'd ask for a bit more. A Buddhist is someone who primarily considers the Buddha to be one's guiding light, and secondly, is convinced that his teachings best help explain ourselves and our world.

These teachings are:

- *Suffering is the common condition of all sentient beings.*
- *Nothing stays unchanged.*
- *"Soul" is a fiction of the human imagination, self-created to deny such change.*
- *"God," too, is a fiction of the human imagination, to allow for such a soul.*
- *Nothing comes out of nothing, everything being interrelated, which is why there is no God or a first cause.*

- *The only way to end suffering is by forgetting God and being self-reliant.*
- *The way out of suffering is through mind cultivation, which will also help you see these realities through one's mind's eye.*

Buddhists of the world are sure to exhibit a range of commitment on each of these points. But as long as one is convinced of these teachings, one is a Buddhist.

---

1. The coming-of-age religious ritual for boys (but now for girls as well).
2. A seven-candle holder used in Jewish observances.

17

THE BUDDHA THROUGH MODERN
LITERARY EYES

The furore of *The Satanic Verses*[1] brings to mind the treatment of the Buddha in two works of fiction, one originally written by a Swiss writer and translated into English, and the other in Sinhala in Sri Lanka.

There are both parallels and differences between Herman Hesse's ever-so-popular novel, *Siddhartha*, and Rushdie's work.

Both were written in a Western language and published in the West, although Hesse was not born into the faith the book deals with.

If Prophet Mohammed is thinly veiled under the name of Mahamed, Siddhartha is the lay name of the Buddha before his renunciation. The Buddha himself becomes a fictional character at the hands of Hesse. Indeed, the cover of the first English translation of *Siddhartha* in 1951 shows a seated Buddha.

Hesse's character, however, does not match the life of historical Siddhartha in all its detail. Our protagonist, for example, ends up as a ferryman and not a Buddha. But there is little doubt that Hesse had the Buddha's life in mind when he developed his character.

Born to a Kshatriya family (the Buddha was born a prince), Siddhartha leaves home "to join the ascetics," and goes from teacher to teacher. Dissatisfied, he goes on a solitary search.

All this is the life of the Buddha. Even the ferryman is symbolic of the Buddha, the one who found the way to help sentient beings across the ocean of life.

In a clever twist of history, Hesse takes Siddhartha, and his companion Govinda, to the Buddha as his last teacher. Leaving the Buddha, Siddhartha goes on the solitary search, just like the historical Siddhartha did, vowing "I'll conquer myself."

This search, however, takes him on a different course from the historical Siddhartha: to a courtesan who he asks to be his "friend and teacher."

In the course of the psychological transformation from spiritual seeker to prisoner of the senses, Hesse uses the same dream technique as the one that has stirred up the Rushdie controversy:

During the night ... Siddhartha had a dream. He dreamt that Govinda stood before him, in the yellow robe of an ascetic ... He embraced Govinda ... and kissed him. He was no longer Govinda, but a woman, and out of the woman's gown emerged a full breast, and Siddhartha lay there and drank; sweet and strong tasted the milk from her breast. It tasted of woman and man ...

Siddhartha's yearning for the body of his former companion suggests both homosexual and heterosexual tendencies.

This scene, as well as the lengthy encounter with the courtesan (covering a full quarter of the novel), who finds herself with child, can be seen as drawing upon Prince Siddhartha's own lay life of twenty-nine years. He lived in a royal household, entertained by wine and dancing women. He had a wife and a son.

Hesse's portrayal of Siddhartha, no doubt, is an extension of historical Siddhartha's life up to renunciation, but incorporating significant elements of life after renunciation.

Hesse is clearly exploring the human side of the Buddha, through thinly veiled fictional detours.

Just as clearly, all this is offensive to the sensibility of the Buddhist. Enlightenment is characterized as a state beyond a shadow of lust, a complete control of the senses.

Despite the liberties taken of the type that would raise the ire of the devout, Hesse departs from Rushdie in one significant way. He does not treat the Buddha irreverently. Indeed, the protagonist addresses the Buddha as, "O Perfect One."

Yet, Siddhartha challenges him:

You show the world as a complete, unbroken chain ... linked together by cause and effect. ... But ... this unity and logical consequence of all things is broken in one place. Through a small gap there streams into the world of unity something strange, something ... that cannot be demonstrated and proved; that is your doctrine of rising above the world, of salvation.

Siddhartha is challenging here one of the Buddha's most fundamental teachings: Nirvana. The entirety of his teachings thus comes tumbling down. The Buddha is no longer the Perfect One!

Or the All-knowing One, as known to millions of followers. The Buddha responds to the challenge with the words, "You have found a flaw."

Now the Buddha admits to his fallibility!

The Buddha even wishes the departing young Siddhartha well in his search.

Wouldn't all this step on the Buddhist sensibility? A redeeming factor for Hesse is that such a freedom is allowed by the Buddha himself.

In his Discourse to the Kalamas, the Buddha says: "... it is proper that you have a doubt."

He further cautions not to accept anything, even in the faith that "this is our teacher," but only upon personal experience.

Today, after forty years, *Siddhartha* still adorns the shelves of libraries and university course outlines in both the Western and the Buddhist world. But what about when it first hit the bookstores?

As I recollect it, the publication hardly moved a feather in the Buddhist world. Buddhist countries like Sri Lanka, Burma and Thailand were just beginning to enjoy political freedom. The literary elite had had their own education and training in the West, and were perhaps too benumbed to the local culture. For the more sensitive, *Siddhartha* would have been simply a twitch of the decadent West, and something to be ignored!

Where *Siddhartha* found ready acceptance was among the North Americans whose search for an alternative lifestyle ended in the hippie culture.

A closer parallel to the Rushdie furore, however, is the Sinhalese novel written in the early sixties by Sri Lanka's Wickremasingha. *bawa taranaya (Crossing the Ocean of Life)* is the very story of the life of the Buddha.

While Wickremasingha, born and raised a Buddhist, handles the Buddha story fictionally with the same respect that Hesse does, his imagination runs riot in one scene, which cuts to the very core of the Sinhalese Buddhist sensibility.

As in history, the Buddha in Wickremasingha's novel returns to his hometown. Here, he is venerated by his father, nursing mother and the royal retinue with deep respect, but keeping their distance.

His former wife, however, takes the liberty of touching his feet and hugging his legs. Wickremasingha, horror of horrors, portrays the Buddha, the one who spends six full years successfully taming his senses, as being sexually excited!

The author was, of course, like Hesse, exploring the human side of the Buddha here. No reason to take offence, the critic argued. The Buddha does not claim to be anything other than human. Enlightenment was no result of divine intervention but of sheer superhuman effort, open to any and all.

Enlightenment, however, is also the overcoming of ordinary humanness.

The Sinhala critics, journalists and intelligentsia were outraged, as were, of course, Buddhist monks. There were calls to ban the book, and pull it off the racks of bookstores and university libraries. But luckily no effigy burnings or death threats!

Luckily again Sri Lanka was no theocratic state. The multifaith secular government let the matter lie where it should: in the hands of the literary world.

In the end, critical dialogue prevailed. Today, as then, *bawa taranaya* adorns the bookshelves and course lists of universities and high schools.

Author Wickremasingha, too, died the same way he lived – respected as a provocative but mature novelist, a scholar of Buddhism and Sinhalese Buddhist culture, and, most importantly, a humanist.

But why go to Switzerland or Sri Lanka to see how the Buddha has taken kickings and beatings with a smile? A Zen master titles his work, *Dropping Ashes on the Buddha*.

Closer to home, in a restaurant lobby in Toronto, a pot-belly laughing Buddha invites you to a soup named after him!

The last time I tasted it, I thought Perfection had found a home in the hands of the Chef!

---

1. *The Satanic Verses* is a book by the British author, Salman Rushdie. It was regarded as blasphemous and raised ire in the Islamic world. A *fatwa* condemming the author to death was issued by the Iranian spiritual leader in 1989.

18

DO CELEBRATE "TEMPLE DAY"

Some time ago when I was asked as the then President of the Buddhist Council of Canada to provide a list of Buddhist holidays for the Multifaith Calendar[1] published in Vancouver, I created one that was not traditional but has come to be recognized in North America.

I called it Temple Day. In doing this, I wasn't being high-handed or arbitrary. I was simply formalizing a tradition that was already emerging.

Buddhism is one of the fastest growing religions in Canada, showing a 215% increase between 1981 and 1991[2], the year of the last census. There are more than fifty or so temples or groups present in Metro and vicinity today[3].

They fall generally into four categories.

Tibetan you perhaps know the best, thanks to the Chinese invasion and the Dalai Lama. The older among us may be more familiar with Zen – the spiritual heart-throb of the flower children of the '60s. Today in Metro, followers are primarily of Japanese, Korean and Vietnamese origins. Chinese Buddhism – from mainland China, Hong Kong and Taiwan – has perhaps the most dynamic growth. Theravada Buddhists, the earliest tradition, are from Sri Lanka, Burma, Cambodia, Laos, with Sinhalese Buddhism (of Sri Lanka) being the oldest of the oldest, dating back 2,300 years.

So what has Temple Day got to do with all of this? It is that whatever the cultural or geographic origin, or skin colour, all Buddhists, or certainly most of them, have made it a practice to go to the temple on the first day of the New Year.

For sure they all have their special days throughout

the year specific to their own form of practice, but they have come to consider the very first holiday of the year a good time to rejuvenate their spiritual energy in whatever way they've decided to do it over the centuries.

It is this fact – the presence of Buddhists of all schools at their temples on this day – that gave legitimacy to Temple Day.

So what do Buddhists do when they go to their temple?

Universally, you will find some form of offering to the Buddha – flowers, incense, candles, fruits, food and medicinal herbs on an altar.

If you are wondering about the medicinal herbs, you perhaps know that the ordained monks and nuns have few personal possessions, no relations and no homes to live in. They are basically dependent on the community. So the Buddha had their health in mind when he suggested medicine to be included as an offering.

You may also hear and see some form of chanting at the temple. This is not to be mistaken as a prayer to the Buddha, although it may come close to it in a few traditions.

You will see worshippers doing five things.

First, they take refuge in the Buddha, *Dhamma* (the teachings) and *Sangha* (the ordained).

Second, they vow to themselves (there is no God in Buddhism) that they will be guided by five training principles: to abstain from taking life, from taking what is not given, from harmful language (lying, slander, back-biting, gossip, etc.), from sexual misconduct and from taking intoxicants to an extent that would alter consciousness.

Third, they offer verbally what is on the altar – to the historical Buddha or to mystical past or future ones.

Fourth, you will find them transferring merit to the departed. You see, doing a good thing has a double dividend – first for doing the good and then for sharing it with others!

Finally, you will find some form of meditation – sitting or walking, quietly or out loud.

So then, if you are not tired after midnight mass or all-night dancing, you might want to drop by a temple of your choice on January 1. Are visitors welcome? You bet! For locations, try the Internet.

See you around on Temple Day. Merry Christmas and Happy New Year![3]

---

1. Published by the Multifaith Action Society and can be ordered through mfcalendar@pacificcoast.net.
2. In 2004 there were over seventy Buddhist organizations in Metro Toronto (buddhismcanada.com). Between the 1991 and 2001 censuses, Buddhism showed a 183% increase.
3. The piece published in December 1996.

19

WE ALL NEED TO REPAY KINDNESSES

Some 2,500 years ago, the Buddha is said to have spent a whole week gazing at the tree that gave him shade as he underwent the Enlightenment experience. Fact or fiction, this little story underscores the place of gratitude in the Buddha's Teachings.

Growing up as kids, we paid homage to our parents – our mothers for "bearing me in the womb ... and nourishing me" and to our fathers for "helping me grow." We wished them long life, too.

A British sociologist writes how, in Sri Lanka, two litigants were seen to work together in the same field, one returning a favour received from the other in his field, before going to court. A living example of societal reciprocity, she commented.

Having just completed the triple celebration of Wesak – the Buddha's birth, Enlightenment and final demise – these thoughts come to mind as I think of the Canadian Red Cross Society, which is now being accused of negligence over HIV-tainted blood.

If, as has been claimed, the venerable institution was less than responsible, it needs to be called to answer. But in doing so, should we abandon a sense of gratitude for the thousands of lives saved for every life affected, or lost, due to blood contamination?

Then there is the June Callwood case. A *Saturday Night* piece allows for the possibility of some lack of judgement on the part of Callwood in handling the case of Nellie's Hostel (in Toronto). When a black woman tried to hand her a flyer as she was leaving Roy Thomson Hall after a PEN meeting, it was discourteous and certainly not becoming of one who has come to be seen as a national treasure, to say "F--- off." Only later would she know the woman herself was a writer – Marlene Nourbese Philips, author of *Harriet's Daughter*. Then there was Callwood's breach of confidentiality of someone who had benefited from Nellie's Hostel but was now an accuser.

The fast conclusion one could arrive at is that Callwood is an "intentional racist." But, given her track record, could she rather not be seen as being a *victim* of "unintentional racism" that is so much ingrained in society? Or perhaps the attack so overwhelmed her that she had no psychological space to realize that, in a changing, multicultural society, the "I'm beyond reproach" attitude she is said to have held could result in racism.

But where is an attempt by the accusers to look at the contributions made by Callwood all these years? Without her, there would be no Nellie's!

Finally, the Masters case. If, as an inquiry concluded, Carlton Masters was sexually offensive to his women staff when he was Ontario's agent-general to the United States, he deserved punishment.

But the more relevant question is whether there was any consideration of the fact that his appointment was one attempt by a government to bring some semblance of balance for which women themselves have been working hard? Was there any concern for this social good in anybody's mind?

These stories are perhaps signs of a larger social malaise – that we are no different today from the self-centred generation of the '60s we mockingly labelled the "me-generation."

I haven't heard one politician, public figure, doctor or nurse defend the Red Cross. Or any human rights, multicultural or feminist voice coming to the help of a beleaguered government, or pinning a laurel on society for allowing the Masters appointment to happen.

We may not need to pay homage at anyone's feet as we did in Sri Lanka as kids. But maybe, like the Buddha, each of us needs to take a minute or two every day, to simply gaze at each other in wonderment, with a deep sense of gratitude, for all the wonderful things we do for each other.

Perhaps we need to ask how we may pay in kind for what everybody else gives to make our lives what they are.

As the Buddha reminds us, hatred begets hatred.

20

DHARMA DAY MESSAGE IS MODERATION

Ears alert, the fawn dashed to the mother as it heard the footsteps of the stranger. Five men in their thirties or forties continued ascetic silence, in a grove called Deer Park, in Benares, India.

The fawn, comforted by the mother who sensed no harm from the approaching stranger, frolicked, attracting more deer, who nosed each other playfully. One of the men turned toward the footsteps, but then returned quickly to his ascetic practice.

The deer pranced as if in anticipation. A second ascetic, answering to the light breeze nudging his bare skin, allowed himself to gaze in the direction of the footsteps. Taken aback but looking closely, he declared, "Oh, it's Gotama."

"Gotama? No doubt he's found himself heading into spiritual wilderness ... Pity he didn't stick with us and the well-worn ascetic path," replied another.

"Let's ignore him," dared a third, to everybody's assent.

But as the quickening breeze enveloped their bodies, the men saw their resolve melt away like snow in the rising sun. Their crossed legs unfolding, one by one, they stood up, although none felt brave enough to let out the feeling of "Wow" welling up within themselves in the majestic presence of their former partner-in-asceticism.

Finally, the lips of the eldest of the Group of Five parted, saying, "Welcome back, Gotama."

"Address me not thus," came the confident words from the smiling face, "you're talking to the Enlightened One."

"Haven't we heard this one," was their reply, although they must have felt they should say, "The Buddha?"

Yes, the Buddha, the one who has eschewed the two extremes.

As if overhearing the exchange, the deer gathered to bear witness to the unfolding of a great event, "The Turning of the Wheel of Dharma," as the ancient text, the *Tipitaka*, puts it.

The five now seated in front of him cross-legged, the Buddha continued, answering his own question, "What two extremes?" The first – "that which is among passions, practicing the enjoyment of passions, inferior, vulgar, common, barbarian ..."

No surprise there, the celibate group concurred, knowing also the life of wine and women Prince Siddhartha, the future Buddha, had spent before taking to the ascetic life.

But the next extreme, that was something else: "that which is devoted to weariness of oneself, unhappy, barbarian ..."

This "weariness of oneself" was the extreme asceticism that he himself had practiced with the Group, and was their continuing spiritual bread and butter! How could they bear to hear their ideal practice condemned as barbarian?

But what they didn't know was that Gotama, upon leaving them, had taken the asceticism to its edges. Frustrated at his failure in gaining liberation from the chain of life (*samsara*), he had not only completely given up eating but had also almost stopped breathing in the thought that it, too, was a form of nutriment, and that it was this gratification of the body that was impeding liberation.

He had given up this extreme practice just in the nick of time to save his life, he explained.

Unconvinced, the Group of Five listened to the

Buddha explain how he then returned to normal living and mastered the art of bringing peace and calm within himself through systematic mind-training. It was during this process that he came to understand the problem with extremes. Both were forms of attachment! Wanting to gratify the senses is an attachment as is wanting to deny the senses of such gratification.

The Middle Path emerged as a natural result.

The deer pranced around in glee, and the wind pirouetted. "Light has dawned, and insight," came the cry, from one, two or more of the Group, their attachment to extremes losing its vigour.

It is this event, this Turning of the Wheel, that Buddhists celebrate in July. It is listed in the Canadian Multifaith Calendar as Dharma Day. Canada will no doubt understand and join in, just as we finish celebrating Canada Day.

21

WHAT WOULD THE BUDDHA SEE AT GENERAL MOTORS?

You leave home for a few days and soon the words come out: "Oh, how I miss my bed!"

Perhaps you've spent a fortune on your bed and it is so comfy. That may be why you miss it.

Or is it? Surely the bed in your hotel room is no less firm or no smaller, and the linen is just as clean. So is it possible there is another reason?

Maybe your mindbody cells – zillions of them – can tell the difference, that the hotel bed gives a very different sensation. And so they have to make an adjustment: "Hey, man, this hurts ... I don't like it one bit!"

How about when your spouse suggests the family should be looking for a different place to live? Or when your company transfers you to a different city? Do you say: "Oh, how I hate to move"?

All these are what could be called "pain of change." So when you fall sick, is it "pain of suffering?"

Those are two kinds of pain we all recognize. So, is it being negative to point out that they are a reality? This is what the Pope, in his bestseller, seems to be saying about the Buddha's teachings.

The Buddha's first "Noble Truth" is *dukkha*, which is of three types.

"Pain of suffering" is one. This refers to the ordinary miseries of life: falling sick, working for that boss, parting company with a loved one (say at death), even being born into the life cycle.

A second is "pain of change." By that, the Buddha means more than just missing your bed – those cells that keep an eye on you, the bundles of atoms of which our bodies are made, are changing before we can bat an eyelid. And the mind is changing even faster, rendering thoughts into a "stream of consciousness," a continuous flow.

As to the third meaning, one might say: "Because the zillions of cells in our mindbody keep changing at this frantic pace, our psyches seem always to feel in a state of instability." But let's get real here. Who wants to feel swept off their feet all the time? So we cheat ourselves with the idea that, "Hey, I'm stable ... I have something that doesn't change and is in charge of the operation."

We even give it a name: soul. And we link it to God.

Because this is a created lie, I call it "reconstructed pain."

I can hear the Buddha, ever the great communicator, now inviting us to the General Motors factory in Oshawa to explain this third "pain."

We first look at the fleet lined up ("Cars, aren't they?")

Then we watch the assembly line. A chassis arrives. An engine is lowered. Joe Mechanic tightens the screws. A carburettor appears. Then some wires. Another piece and another. Seats go into place. Then the body is lowered. And finally, the wheels are put on.

The Buddha then puts the key into the ignition switch and the engine roars. Everybody claps. Over the hum, the Buddha asks: "What is a Car?"

Everybody scrambles for an answer. But Ms Sharp says: "Yeah, I see. It is nothing but the sum of its total parts. There is no single part that keeps the car going. It is all the parts working together in tandem."

"Bravo, Ms Sharp. I couldn't have put it better ... The 'car' is our 'mindbody.' Its 'electrical energy' is our psychic energy that we call 'the mind.' Like you said, there is nothing, apart from its parts, that controls the running of the car. The car is the parts, the parts the car."

"But why is all this a pain, sir?"

"Because it blinds us to the reality of 'things as they are.' It is this ignorance, or self-cheating, that keeps us going in this life cycle. And because we're blinded, we can't find a solution.

"This is all I meant 2,500 years ago, and I mean now.

"Meditate upon it," the Buddha says with a smile, as we wave goodbye.

22

BARE-BREAST IMAGE STAYS IN MEMORY

Bare-breasts on the street. Tobacco ads. Crime on celluloid.

What do these have in common? Nothing perhaps, except they have all been news items in the last few months. But there is, indeed, something, from a Buddhist point of view.

The judge acquitting the woman who went bare-breasted on the street one summer day said, "No one who was offended was forced to continue looking at her."

The tobacco industry argues that its ads don't add to the rise in smoking among teenagers.

And a *Toronto Star* front page story on June 23, 1996, headlined: "Don't blame TV for Violence: Experts".

All three arguments are dead wrong, not for moral or social reasons, but for psychological ones.

The Buddha explains how our senses work in terms of three conditions. Taking the example of what he calls eye consciousness, he gives the first two conditions as (1) a working physical eye and (2) a working mental eye or an eye-door path to the brain. So far, this is basic psychology that we all know, only using the language of 2,500 years ago.

We can think of Helen Keller as a twentieth-century example. When her mom waved her hand or shone a bright light in front of her eyes on that fateful day when Helen went blind, the girl simply stared straight ahead. She had a physical eye, but her mental eye wasn't working.

Condition (3) is stimulus. This, too, is basic psychology – except that the Buddha would say that it, too, is part of the perceiver's eye-consciousness; it is not something just sitting outside of you.

But, of course Helen's mom's hand was for real; only it just wasn't part of Helen's world.

There is a parallel process for ear-, nose-, tongue- and body-consciousness.

If that is how consciousness works, taking your eyes off the bare breasts you've just seen on the street wouldn't make one bit of a difference to the person – psychologically. You may be able to show your respect for the woman's right to bare herself, but by the time you take your eyes off, it is already part of your consciousness.

This happens because now the Buddha's sixth sense, mind-consciousness, kicks in and in high gear! The mental image now acts as stimulus, and so the bare-breast consciousness continues to linger, in memory.

The tobacco ad on TV or the crime scene on the screen would likewise etch in a memory – as smoking-consciousness, violence-consciousness, etc.

By itself such a memory may be harmless. However, there are the associations. So, if we were to see in an ad someone lighting up at a party, the party becomes another of the conditions of the eye-consciousness. And for the young who don't have the life experiences to tell you otherwise, smoking becomes part of fun-consciousness. Respectable and authority-challenging, too! The warning on the pack is less likely to become a stimulus for consciousness because it is not associated with fun.

Bare breasts on the street similarly come to be associated not just with the innocent need for a whiff of cool air. Remember, we are a society promoting sexuality, with the cunning, if not the venom and the persistence, of a Trojan horse, and with male ad designers baring breasts to sell products rather than to highlight sexuality and potential violence against women.

"It's violence in the... mind not on the television screen that sparks a violent act," the Star article says. But what the experts don't say is how violence came to be in the mind in the first place. Couldn't the watching of violence on screen trigger that latent karmic potential into action?

The Buddha's idea that stimulus is part of consciousness puts the onus on us to think about how we put our stimuli on show – be it body parts, behaviours, ideas or values.

23

TEN PATHS LEAD TO PERFECTION

Want to be perfect, living in this imperfect world? Try the Buddhist Perfections (*parami* or *paramita*). They are basically virtues, cultivated with compassion but guided by reason and are not based on selfish conceit. Here is the checklist of Ten Perfections (in a slightly changed order). See how you fare, grading yourself from 1 to 4.

1. *Loving-kindness*: If you think friendliness to your best friend, you have the idea. A score of 1 would be "friendly to yourself," of 2, "to your immediate family," of 3, "to the country or world you live in," and 4, "to all sentient beings and nature."

2. *Sharing* or *generosity*: One of the most highly valued practices in the Buddhist world, this is the idea of sharing whatever goodies, material or other. A smile, a good meal, happiness – all count. Score 1 would be "me, me" and 4, "the wide world."

3. *Self-discipline*: Isn't this what every parent, teacher, religion asks of you? In Buddhist daily practice, this would be in relation to five abstinences: from killing, stealing, sensual misbehaviour, lying and intoxicants. Killing includes animals and insects, and intoxicants to an extent that alters consciousness. Give yourself 1 for "seldom abstaining from any one of them" and a 4 for "always, for all five."

4. *Wisdom*: *Buddha* means the Knowing One. His Enlightenment meant understanding reality as it is. But knowing facts is not wisdom. Wisdom results from a compassionate attitude. A high score of 4 is when facts are synthesized to allow a holistic picture and are linked with a moral base.

5. *Effort* or *energy*: We know this almost by osmosis.

It is all around us. Put some energy into it, sports coaches and bosses tell us. You get marks for effort at school. A 1 rating is for "little effort," and a 4 for "as much as I can."

6. *Patience*: What scientists bring to their work and what you have by the bushel at the doctor's office. But what you don't have waiting at a red light or when things don't go your way. You get a 1 for "rarely" and a 4 for "always in everything."

7. *Truthfulness*: You won't be tolerated in the courts if you don't swear/affirm to tell the truth and nothing but the truth. And if as kids, we lied at school and got caught, we know how quickly we ended up in the principal's office. Give yourself 1 for "never, if I can get away with it," and 4 for "never, if I can at all help it."

8. *Determination*: Just look at where you are and how you got there. Could you have done it without determination – getting an education, keeping a clean home and environment, getting that promotion, buying that first home or car? Now by contrast, you may want to think of how you or someone you know didn't get somewhere you or he wanted to. "Little determination" gets a 1 and "the story of your life" rates a 4.

9. *Equanimity*: This is possibly a uniquely Buddhist value. The basic idea is not to allow yourself to be on a yo-yo – going up at success and down in failure. The higher the excitement at success or gain, the higher the misery in failure or loss. So the trick, the Buddha says, is to keep your cool in both situations. To get "excited at the drop of a hat" gets a 1 and to "stay calm and cool at any and everything," a 4.

10. *Renunciation*: It sounds like leaving home to live the life of an ascetic and celibate. It is, if you are into that world-renouncing mode. But as we live in the world, it can mean "renouncing an ice cream" for a 1 or "giving up booze" for a 4.

Now post the list on your fridge for future use and add up the total, and you will know how perfect you are ...

24

MEDITATION ERASES FEAR OF DEATH

Both the Buddha and Freud must be dead wrong. Dead, for sure! But wrong? Freud talks of *thanatos* – the death instinct. And the Buddha talks of the "thirst to be not."

It was with these thoughts that I wrote an earlier column on organ transplantation[1] in which I made a plea to please consider donating body parts for transplantation so that another could live. I had assumed that death is part of life, and therefore that death would be boldly faced as we face life.

I also invited readers to share with me if they had any reservations, religious or otherwise. To my amazement, no response.

So, I'm trying to figure out why. Is it that, metaphysically, we humans perhaps have no innate thirst, or instinct, to die as the Buddha and Freud would have us believe? Or is it that, as a North American Buddhist friend tells me, "a pornography of death" is making the rounds? It appears mum's the word, in our youth-loving culture, when it comes to death.

This is so, no doubt, for very good reasons. But talking about it, Buddhists believe, can make a world of difference.

"Life constituents are of the nature of decay. Arising and decay are their reality. Having arisen they decay. May these (thoughts) bring you relief and comfort," a Buddhist is reminded at funeral services.

Hobnobbing with death, then, can prepare you for when that inevitable event arrives – like an athlete practicing until the Olympics arrive. Going through the strain, repeatedly, makes it familiar territory. The same is true, Buddhism holds, when it comes to death.

So how can one make death familiar territory? By visiting it, of course, ahead of time, again and again. Through meditation.

One may begin by trying to understand what death is. Doesn't knowledge set you free?

So, what, then, is death?

Death is a mere extended period of a process that we experience every moment. In living, we breathe in and then breathe out. The breath comes to be and passes away. Now imagine that we don't breathe in again. That is all that death is. Not breathing. Not taking in that next breath. The body has no energy to draw that fresh air.

But what is that body that has no strength to take in that breath? A meditation reminds us:

There is in this body head hair, body hair, nails, teeth, skin, flesh, sinews, bone, marrow, kidneys, heart, liver, pleura, spleen, lungs, intestines, mesentery, stomach, feces, bile, phlegm, pus, blood, sweat, solid fat, tears, liquid fat, saliva, mucus, synovic fluid, urine and a brain in a skull.

The purpose here, of course, is to reflect upon a simple fact – body is nothing but the sum of its (32) parts. And, like the breath, each of them, too, has the nature of coming to be and passing away.

With that awareness in mind, a practitioner of meditation is encouraged to take the next step – visualize one's own full body. Then, lie flat on the back, letting out that breath that you took last and not taking in the next. In the mind's eye, you're now lying there still. And cold.

Next, the body is no more, only a skeleton. (To help with this visualization, one may have a skeleton, as I do, of a type used in medical labs.) Soon, one visualizes a skeleton reduced to individual bones, all finally turned to powder.

At the beginning of any, or all, of these meditations, of course, there may possibly be great psychological discomfort, as with anything new. But with time, and practice, the mind will begin to accept the reality of death, in its different stages.

Having then visited the realm of death, as the end of breathing, the body turned skeleton, bones and ashes, it brings no surprises when it finally hits. Fear taken out, through meditation and reflection, one is more ready to face it.

Calmly.

---

1. See chapter 5.

25

EUTHANASIA MAY BE A HEALING WELL-DEATH

The word "euthanasia" is made up of *eu* and *thanatos*, literally "well" plus "death" in Greek. And our present emphasis seems to be on the death dimension of the formula.

On this basis, Buddhism would also say that terminating life, either your own or another, is clearly a violation of the first precept of "not taking life." But "the middle path" as advocated by the Buddha can bring some balance to the scales.

Here then is one leg of that balance: the *intent* of the act of killing, about which the Buddha's words are, "Intent, I say, is *karma*."

You know what karma is all about, don't you? It is what you pay for in a next life for being naughty or nice in this life. Or what you pay for in this life for your commissions or transgressions in a previous life. Right?

Yes, but in the quoted context, it also means "action." Simply any action. So if the intent of the action was *not* killing, but rather the *alleviation of suffering*, then there may not be a violation of the precept.

Now to the other leg – the outcome of the resulting death – what else is the *outcome* of death other than death itself?

Ah, but the Buddhist views death as but one scene of a continuing drama, a temporary stopover in an ongoing samsaric cycle of lives. There is always a second, third ... nay, a multitude of chances to get your act together. The Buddha had 548, the texts say!

In this light, killing (better, helping to die) again comes to be alleviating suffering in this life. Isn't that amazing, the coming together of the two legs?

With both intent and outcome, the action of helping to die comes not within the range of criminal activity but within the range of healing activity – one extreme beginning with taking an aspirin for a headache, and the other, having the heart stopped momentarily in a heart transplant. In a "well-death," that would be having the heart stopped for a longer time, say until consciousness finds a new home in a new "mindbody."

Helping to die to alleviate pain, then, is an act of compassion – to help the afflicted find a new, and hopefully better, home. It is another opportunity to snap out of a past karmic misery.

Focusing exclusively on the death segment of the euthanasia formula puts us into a legal straitjacket; focusing on the healing side directs our mind to the spiritual life chance.

This is all theory, fine and dandy, you would say, but what would you do if you had Lou Gehrig's disease or some such horrible thing?

Naturally, it would depend on the stage of my disease and the severity of my pain, but all things considered, my preference, I think, will be to live through my illness as long as I can. But, no machines please.

If my practice (of meditation) were strong enough to bring out the compassion in me, part of my consideration would be the suffering of my loved ones.

Now what if I were a Buddhist health professional? My first and most persistent recommendation would be for hospice care – including, ideally, daily sessions of meditation, to calm the mind. But with repeated requests from the afflicted, and in the absence of any alternatives, I might agree to assisting. This, of course, not forgetting the consequences, in terms of karmic reaction and social implications.

What if I were a Buddhist legislator in the House of

Commons? I would take the floor to argue that euthanasia has nothing to do with the law and that it should be the responsibility of the afflicted, or someone responsible, in consultation with health professional(s) if need be. And that it would be up to the governing body of the given profession to pass judgement on the professional concerned.

And as a citizen, or a community member, I would offer to sit in meditation with the affected family.

26

WOULD EUTHANASIA HINDER REBIRTH?

In the earlier column on euthanasia, which I called "well-death" on the basis of etymology, I wrote about the need to balance the "death" and "well" components.

Linking a karma element – i.e., consequences of our past or present behaviour in terms of the three doors of mind, body and language – I made the point that, if euthanasia is well-intentioned, bad consequences would not accrue to the one who mediates.

For the same reason, it should not be considered murder, from the legal point of view, either.

While this point is still valid, I would like now to look at the issue in relation to the person subjected to euthanasia.

Again, karma enters the picture, remembering the Buddhist understanding of a *samsara* lifecycle. In each birth we carry the memories of those past lives.

It would be obvious from the point of view of karma that a handicap or horrific illness could be understood as a fruition of karma.

Such a scenario becomes even more complex when we consider the Buddhist teaching relating to the realms of existence. There are six in number. Life as a human being, of course, is only one of them, and we know the second – as an animal.

But if these are the only two in which both mind and body come to be manifested, there are four more where only the mind energy lives on. We may think of it as "life between life" or post-death, pre-birth "interlife," or as in Tibetan Buddhism, "*bardo*."

To be (re)born as a "shining one," or *deva*, in one of the "upper" two realms, is to experience a happy living.

But not so in the two "lower" realms. Popular religion tells us what it means to be born as a "hell-being"; it is simply sheer hell. But to be born as a "hungry ghost" is to be always hungry, always trying to survive!

As in physics, every action has an equal reaction.

To point to this is not to point fingers or to minimize our sympathy, but to remind ourselves of reality.

If a handicap or chronic illness is then a "working off" of one's karma, then euthanasia may be, in fact, an unkind intervention. For it might mean that the sentient being might need one or more births to complete the "unfinished business."

The working of karmic memory is such that we simply don't know if, indeed, one will be born into one of the two miserable realms. But unfinished business resulting from euthanasia just might be a condition for such a rebirth. Finishing off the business in this life, on the other hand, may be a way of avoiding it.

Again we have to be careful to remind ourselves that this is not a threat of damnation, but simply the working of genetic memory.

So would euthanasia maximize or minimize the chances for a human rebirth? Death in Buddhism I called "exit-consciousness" and birth, "relinking consciousness." What this suggests is the close relationship between the two. Dying of natural causes, of course, would allow for the most peaceful form of exit-consciousness. Euthanasic intervention, on the other hand, may traumatize the natural exit process. Would this be a condition for rebirth in a lower realm? We can only conjecture.

So am I against euthanasia? In my earlier column I may have sounded like I am for it. But all I am doing here is pointing out the other dimension.

So is it a cop-out? Not at all. Which particular course of action I personally would take, as an afflicted person or an intervener, would depend on my state of spirituality at the time.

Until then, all I can do is keep working on my own spirituality so that, hopefully, it will help me arrive at that critical decision.

27

IN DEATH, WE ARE ALL UNITED

There is nothing but death that doth remind us of death. Recently, I got a jolt twice: one, a family member in a far away land, the other, a long time family friend in Toronto.

I hadn't had much contact with either of them over the years, yet both brought home a sense of my own mortality and with it, what one could do for a dying dear one.

It was after my friend fell into a coma that I came to know that an ulcer had decided to keep him company. Now it had him in its grip, like a tropical python, taking him toward what the Buddha calls the "exit-mind."

That meant that he still had a mind – a working mind – however dead it may appear to us. To my Buddhist way of thinking, he was then not *un*conscious but *sub*-conscious, which meant I could still communicate with my friend, man to man, one last time!

When I entered his room at home, where he had decided to die, he lay on his bed, face turned to his side. The IV line dangling from a stand was his only sustenance and treatment. At his bedside were the nurse and his wife, son and daughter.

I sat beside him, and called his name, putting my palm on his forehead, stroking. I said my name, and started talking.

"Do you remember the good times we had together ... laughing, chatting ... when you had my daughter on your lap, and I had yours on mine? How we enjoyed a cup of tea over jokes, and shared stories of growing up?"

There was nary a response. But I continued to talk of other good times our two families had had.

I prompted him to think of his many good deeds, such as being one of the few who helped up front with money to purchase a building for the temple.

I watched in silence, allowing him space to swim in his good thoughts and deeds, on his own time ...

Then I reminded him what kind of head of family he had been. "The test of the pudding is in the eating, isn't it?" I said. "Look at your children. Well educated, and professionals, with a future assured ... What more can you ask?"

"Hey, man, you've got a million dollar family. Both settled into family life, too," I reminded him. "Your wife also has her own professional involvement."

I watched, letting my words sink in. Still stroking his forehead, I now turned to religion.

"Yes, my friend, you've accrued a lot of merit – worked as a professional, gave company to a loving wife, helped raise a family, contributed to the community. But now, my friend, it is time to let go ... to unhook from this life ..."

"So begin to think of your next life, leading your 'exit-mind' toward the 'conception-mind' to guide it with the same gentleness you did this life ..."

"Let go, let go, let go."

Continuing to stroke his forehead, I chanted the lines from the Friendliness Discourse. Then I said, "I am not going to say good-bye to you, my friend. I'll leave that to you to do, whenever you're ready."

Holding his hand, I waited. His chest heaved, three times. Had he heard me? Or was it just a coincidence? Does it matter?

But what does matter was that I had had a similar experience with a Christian colleague. He had been hit with a disease that saw him die within weeks. I saw him when he was conscious. And, with his permission and that of the family, I whispered in his ear the same words, with minor variations, as for my Buddhist friend. And we talked about it.

He, a professor of systematic theology, asked me to come to his bedside, again, in his dying hours. I followed the same sequence – personal relationship, family, community, good times and then letting go, of this life, preparing for the next.

His chest didn't heave. But when he passed away, I broke bread with the family and friends, in the name of Jesus. A new experience to me, but I wondered: doth mankind need death to unite us?

28

BUDDHIST STORY PUTS DEATH IN PERSPECTIVE

Recently, disaster struck a woman known to us. She lost both her mother and her only child in an accident.

As my wife and I embraced the young mother at the funeral home, I began to sob, out loud.

I had tried hard to contain my feelings. But I believe my weeping gave the woman, also a professional, permission to give public vent to her feelings.

I don't know about her, but I sure felt good. I'm glad I could cry the way I did when, in another time and place, my own mother's coffin was shut for the last time. I'm glad I didn't feel compelled to follow the convention, especially for men, not to cry in public.

As I reflect on our friend's tragedy, a story well known in Buddhist literature comes to mind. It is the tale of Kisagotami, who loses her only son, who dies when he was just a toddler.

Stricken with grief, she carries the dead body of her son, and goes around looking for medicine that would restore him. People thought she was mad, but advised by a wise man, she comes by the Buddha, asking that he bring her child back to life. He tells her to get a mustard seed from a house in the village that has never had a death in it.

You guessed it. She did not have to come back to the Buddha to cure her anguish. By the end of her futile search, reality had dawned – the reality that death is the common thread to one and all.

The Buddha, of course, had expected this result in sending her on the errand.

Kisagotami's search and discovery led her to become

a disciple of the Buddha and to meditate on the fleeting nature of life.

A monk summoned to a funeral service in a Buddhist family would remind everyone of that thought, and refer to some aspect of *anicca*, the teaching of impermanence.

The grieving family then joins the family leader – husband, wife or oldest child – to pour water into a bowl until it overflows, while the monks chant:

> *Just as a rising river, unto the ocean flows,*
> *rendering it fuller,*
> *May this merit, too (as it overflows), benefit the*
> *departed.*

As the family does this, everyone joins in the thought vibrations. The idea is to share whatever merit one accrues with the dead in order to help them in their sojourn. It is this aspect of a Buddhist funeral that touches me the most.

The event of death, always, leaves me fuller.

I remember that we can help the dead by directing our thoughts to them. The immediacy of my meditation on the fleeting nature of reality is augmented, as I visualize the dead person in its different stages: human to skeleton to dust. My anxiety over my own death is eased in this way.

Why did both grandma and granddaughter have to exit this world at the same time? Perhaps to work out unfinished karmic business together. Like stars, we are reborn in clusters.

It is not difficult to imagine a parent who has died, to be born again, and find a home as a child to a just-wedded daughter. Anyone – grandpa, neighbour, friend or enemy – can be called home, over generations.

29

AN EXERCISE TO OVERCOME
RESENTMENT

Many of us have probably not yet overcome the resentments triggered by the Days of Protest, which pitted not only a "right-wing" government against a "left-wing" citizenry, but also friend against friend. Many of us were tormented by pulls in opposite directions.

Hospital closings, threats by doctors, threats to teachers, talk of amalgamation of the boroughs into a megacity, talk of privatizing firefighting, and attempts at putting the welfare and refugee houses in order may also be adding to the tension.

All this, no doubt, has brought anger, enmity and stress within us.

Let us, then, see if we can do some healing so that we can keep our inner calm, and be "a rock unmoved in the wildest hurricane," to quote a line from the popular Buddhist work, the *Dhammapada*.

Toward this end, then, let us try some Friendliness Meditation, *Metta Bhavana*. The lines are very simple:

May I be free from enmity,
May I be free from ill-will,
May I be free from distress,
May I keep myself happy.

Begin by thinking of yourself as your own friend. Think of the last time you were happy and keep that as the focus of your attention for as long as you can.

Smile if you can, as you keep your eyes fully closed or partly open (with eyes no more than about a metre in front of you). If your attention goes elsewhere, acknowledge it – this is important. Acknowledge it and gently remind yourself that you were with your smile and your happiness, and return to it. Say the words out loud if you like.

Next think of someone not related to you but who has made a difference in your life.

Now say the four lines inserting his/her name, remembering why s/he is important to you. If bad things about the person come to your mind, acknowledge them. But remind yourself that you were looking at why the persons is important to you.

Now think of a dear friend. This should be easy enough. Extend your friendliness to this and return.

Next think of a neutral person – bank teller, postie, bus driver, the person who walks past your house with a dog on a leash, and so on, someone with whom you have no personal relationship but encounter all the time. Repeat the four lines in relation to that person. Acknowledge any distraction and return.

By this time, already about twelve to twenty minutes (if not longer) into it, and with experience, your mind will be expanded by a pervasive sense of friendliness.

This expansion will make the next step much easier – to extend your *metta* to someone who eats into you – at work, among relatives and acquaintances, your competition.

Now, close your eyes, if necessary, and visualize that face. See that rare (or perhaps not so rare) smile in that face. Now say the lines in relations to him/her. As earlier, acknowledge any distractions and return.

Now, after a few minutes of this meditation, and at the end of the series, visualize the faces of all of the people you have thought of, placing them alongside your own. See their smiles.

Now extend the Friendliness Meditation to one and

all, beginning with yourself and ending with the unloved one. Do it in forward and reverse order, several times over. Acknowledge any distraction and return.

The goal of this part of the practice, of course, is to cultivate equanimity, an egalitarianism, putting everybody on a par.

But if your think Friendliness Meditation is pure altruism, think again. Many are the benefits that accrue to your own well-being. If nothing else, you should be sleeping well, and waking up well. It will help you push those negative emotions away and keep within yourself a sense of happiness.

If you keep up the practice throughout your life, say the texts, one dies unconfused. Now wouldn't that be incentive enough?

GLOSSARY

Anatta—literally "not self." The quality of all phenomena that they have no independent core or self. One of the three marks. Everything that exists is influenced by everything else. Nothing can ever stand alone.

Anicca—transience. The quality of all phenomena that they are subject to decay and dissolution.

Asoulity—a translation of *anatta*—the quality of all phenomena that they have no independent core or soul.

Attachment—psychological dependence on the existence of some object or idea.

Bhikkhu—a Buddhist monk

Bhikkhuni—a Buddhist nun

Buddhadharma—the teaching of the Buddha

Dhamma—The teaching, *Dhamma* is the Pali. Dharma is the term in Sanskrit.

Dukkha—suffering, unsatisfactoriness, the quality of all phenomena that it is incapable of producing lasting satisfaction. It is interrelated with *anatta* and *anicca*, for that which is transient cannot provide satisfaction that lasts, and that which has no self, cannot be relied upon to stay the same. It is *dukkha* that the meditator is attempting to overcome. Cessation of *dukkha* is the goal of the Buddha's path.

Enlightenment—the realization of *nibbana:* the sure knowledge that everything is perfect as it is. It is a realization that cannot be described in words. The Buddha typically described it in negative terms, e.g., the end of craving and hatred, the end of suffering, the end of birth and death. It can also be seen as the highest happiness, the deepest peace. It is the goal to which the Buddha's path leads.

Five aggregates—five aspects of mind and body that make up the whole of human experience. The five are materiality, feeling, perception, mental formations and consciousness. The Buddha used this kind of breakdown to point out that each of these elements of experience is incapable of producing lasting happiness.

Karma—Literally "action.," *karma* is used to denote the fact that actions in the ethical realm, have results in kind. Wholesome actions lead to pleasant resultants (e.g., generosity leading to riches) and unwholesome actions lead to unpleasant resultants (e.g., theft leading to poverty).

Lovingkindness—see *Metta*

Metta—lovingkindness, goodwill, friendliness. The wholesome attitude of mind that wants a person or being to be happy and well. The love of a mother for a child. There are specific meditations in the Buddhist teaching that encourage the growth of this attitude.

Nibbana—literally "cessation." The Buddha used this term to denote Enlightenment, the cessation of craving, hatred and attachment, and those conditions that necessitate rebirth and the continuation of the round of suffering.

Nirvana—Sanskrit for *nibbana*. See *nibbana*.

Noble Eightfold Path—a set of eight behavioural and mental factors that need cultivating in order to attain Enlightenment. The eight are right view, right thought, right speech, right action, right livelihood, right effort, right mindfulness and right concentration.

Noble Truth—There are Four Noble Truths, the fundamental teaching of the Buddha. They explain why and how the teaching exists. The Four are: the truth of suffering, the truth of the origin of suffering (which is craving) the truth of the cessation of suffering and the truth of the path leading to the cessation of suffering.

Precepts—the basic ethical constraints asked of followers of the Buddha. These are considered to be rules of training, i.e., their purpose is to help in the search for Enlightenment. Lay people are typically asked to follow five basic precepts: refraining from killing and harming; from taking what is not given; from sexual misconduct; from wrong speech; and from strong drink and intoxicants.

Samsara—the endless round of rebirth. Beings are thought to be reborn in the different realms (human, heavens and hells) according to their actions, until wisdom is developed to the point where Enlightenment arises, and escape from the wheel is possible.

Sangha—the Buddhist community

Tanha—craving. The word literally means *thirst*. The cause of suffering is wanting things to be different from what they are. Craving is a chosen action. The role of the path is to learn when one is craving and to restrain it, thereby reducing and eventually eliminating its unavoidable outcome: suffering.

Three marks—the three marks are three qualities that all phenomena—physical or conceptual—exhibit. They are *dukkha*, or unsatisfactoriness, *anicca* or transience, and *anatta* or non-self.

Vinaya—the code of conduct for the ordained community. In traditional countries, the monks follow 227 rules. Nuns follow these plus an additional 50.

Wesak—Literally the month of May from the ancient Indian Calendar. In Buddhist practice *Wesak* denotes the full moon of that month, a day when the Buddha's birth, Enlightenment and final demise (*paranibbana*) are celebrated.

INDEX

The following books by the same author are available at:

Publisher
Nalanda College of Buddhist Studies
47 Queen's Park Crescent East
Toronto, ON, Canada M5S 2C3
Tel: 416-782-8227 (1-800- if out of town)
E-mail: publisher@nalandacollege.ca.

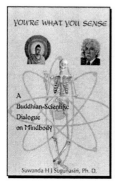 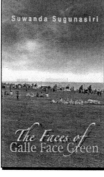 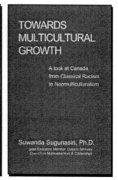

Order Form

Name of Purchaser: _____

Purchase Order No. _____ Date: _____

Address: _____

Tel: _____ E-mail _____

Qty	Item	Price	Total
	Embryo as Person: Buddhism,		
	Bioethics & Society	$ 13.95	
	You're What You Sense:		
	Buddha on Mindbody	$ 19.95	
	The Faces of Galle Face Green		
	(poetry)	$ 11.95	
	Towards Multicultural Growth	$ 19.95	
	Sub-total	$	
	S & H		
	GST		
	TOTAL	$	

☐ Enclosed: Cheque   ☐ Money Order

6 <u>Accept</u> resp'y
10 No Soul, no God
13 - Give organs - why not?
72 - No aggression
36 Homelessness - huh?
40 - God banks - ila
46 - Soul + God - Right change
  - Chastised for Buddh'm - no soul/God
50 - B vs Muslim sacrilege
65 - Not seeing?
  * <u>Have</u> seen!